The Neurologic Patient

The Neurologic Patient

A Nursing Perspective

Sandra DeYoung, R.N., M.A., Ed.M.
Certified Doctoral Candidate, Teachers College,
Columbia University

PRENTICE-HALL, INC., Englewood Cliffs, New Jersey 07632

Library of Congress Cataloging in Publication Data

DeYoung, Sandra.
    The neurologic patient.

    Includes bibliographies and index.
    1. Neurological nursing. I. Title. [DNLM:
1. Neurology—Nursing Texts. 2. Nervous system
diseases—Nursing. WY 160 D529sn]
RC350.5.D48 1983   610.73'68   82-11238
ISBN 0-13-611475-X

*Editorial/production supervision
and interior design by* Maria McKinnon
Cover design by Edsal Enterprises
Manufacturing buyer: John Hall

Printed in the United States of America

10 9 8 7 6 5 4 3 2 1

ISBN 0-13-611475-X

PRENTICE-HALL INTERNATIONAL, INC., *London*
PRENTICE-HALL OF AUSTRALIA PTY. LIMITED, *Sydney*
EDITORA PRENTICE-HALL DO BRASIL, Ltda., *Rio de Janeiro*
PRENTICE-HALL CANADA INC., *Toronto*
PRENTICE-HALL OF INDIA PRIVATE LIMITED, *New Delhi*
PRENTICE-HALL OF JAPAN, INC., *Tokyo*
PRENTICE-HALL OF SOUTHEAST ASIA PTE. LTD., *Singapore*
WHITEHALL BOOKS LIMITED, *Wellington, New Zealand*

Contents

CHAPTER 3   ALTERATIONS IN MOVEMENT   37

CHAPTER 4   ALTERATIONS IN ELIMINATION OF BODY WASTES   70

CHAPTER 5   ALTERATIONS IN RESPIRATORY FUNCTION   87

Preface

In an era in which nursing is trying to identify itself and prove its worth to the public and to other professionals, it is important that nursing textbooks deal with those unique contributions of nursing to the health of the patient. Nursing students and many practicing nurses often have difficulty differentiating between the roles of medicine and nursing, and it isn't surprising. Nursing textbooks which deal primarily with diseases and medical care are apt to mislead the reader into thinking that there is little unique or independent in the realm of nursing.

My approach in this book is to identify, through broad nursing diagnoses, those problems of neurologic patients with which nurses can deal, often independently of medicine. I have avoided exhaustive listing of diseases and have focused instead on common pathological processes involving the nervous system. The nursing problems and concerns which result from the pathology are organized according to the nursing process. Thus, you will see sections on nursing assessment and planning and intervention with evaluation usually interwoven. Examples of specific nursing diagnoses are given at the end of each chapter.

Since neurologic disorders frequently affect every body system and function, I have covered all the major effects in the chapters. You will see from the chapter headings that alterations in nutrition, respiration, and elimination are covered, as well as many other topics; the alterations discussed are only those that result from neurologic disease or injury.

In the first chapter you will find a brief review of anatomy and physiology of the nervous system. This is by no means an extensive coverage of the subject, but it will help you to recall the major structures and functions of the nervous system to enable you to understand the scientific basis of nursing care for neurologic patients.

Terms which are specific to neurology and which may not be familiar to the reader are explained in the text, but for easy reference I have also included a glossary with commonly accepted definitions as I have used them. An appendix incorporating diagnostic tests and nursing implications has been included in chart form. Also in the appendix you will find a chart listing the major neurologic diseases and the nursing problems commonly accompanying those diseases, for quick reference.

My purpose in writing this book is not only to demonstrate that nursing can be defined and separated from other health care disciplines, but also to provide a clear and practical source of information on how to cope with the problems of a neurologic patient using the nursing process. The book will be appropriate for use as a supplementary text for nursing students or as a nursing manual for practicing nurses who deal with neurologic patients and are responsible for planning and carrying out their care.

I wish to thank Gloria Just and Eda Adams for their help in the initial planning of this book and for the continuing support of my family during the writing of it.

Sandra DeYoung

The Neurologic Patient

Review of Anatomy
and Physiology
of the Nervous System

The structure and function of the nervous system are complex and often perplexing to nurses and nursing students. A certain amount of knowledge about the subject is necessary, though, in order to understand the pathology that affects our patients and to provide meaning to our nursing care. This chapter is a review of those aspects of neuroanatomy and neurophysiology which must be grasped in order to provide basic nursing care to neurologic patients. In the rest of the book, further details about anatomy and physiology are included where necessary to increase comprehension of pathology.

FUNCTIONS OF THE NERVOUS SYSTEM

The nervous system enables us to cope with both external and internal environments. The responsiveness of the system to external environmental stimuli permits us to avoid danger, move around in the environment, and interact with other beings. Internal functioning provides a communication network among all body systems, sending, receiving, and interpreting messages that allow us to cope with changes in the internal environment.

Since the nervous system helps to integrate the function of all body systems, a dysfunction in the nervous system can have widespread effects. A problem in the spinal cord, for instance, can result in difficulties in movement, sensation, digestion, elimination, and sexual function. So you can see that to care for a neurologic patient, you have to know the effects of neurologic pathology on the entire body.

Nerve Cells

The basic functioning unit of the nervous system is the nerve cell. It is at this point that all nervous system responsiveness and regulation begins.

The most important of the nerve cells are the *neurons*. The neurons transmit all impulses within the nervous system. They are comprised of a cell body and several projections or nerve fibers. There are several short fibers on one side of the cell body which are called *dendrites* and which bring impulses into the cell body. On the other side of the cell body is one long fiber called the *axon*, which conducts impulses away from the cell body.

Impulses may begin in the brain, brainstem, or from peripheral nerve endings in the skin. These impulses are then usually conducted

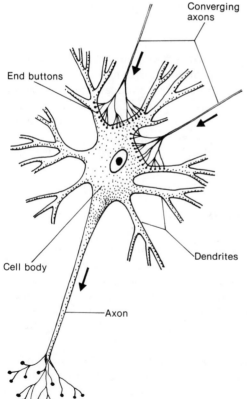

Converging
axons

End buttons

Cell body

Dendrites

Axon

Figure 1.1 Two neurons in synapse with a third neuron. (From William F. Evans, *Anatomy and Physiology*, 2nd ed., ©1976, p. 150. Reprinted by permission of Prentice-Hall, Inc., Englewood Cliffs, N.J.)

over a series of neurons, moving from the axon of one neuron to the dendrites or cell body of the next, eventually reaching an *effector*, an end organ where a response takes place. The effector may be a muscle, an internal organ (including the brain), or a gland. Thus, messages are sent or received by the nervous system, and action is taken accordingly.

The point at which two or more neurons meet (or where a neuron meets a muscle) is called a *synapse* (see Figure 1.1). The axons of one or more neurons come very close to, but do not actually touch, the dendrites or cell body of the next neuron. In most cases, the impulse is conducted across this gap or synapse by a chemical called *acetylcholine*. Then the impulse is inactivated by the enzyme, *cholinesterase*.

One more anatomical feature of neurons that is important to mention is *myelin*. Axons are covered with a white lipid substance called myelin which protects and insulates these fibers. The white myelin gives the name *white matter* to those areas of the brain and spinal cord consisting mostly of myelinated axons. *Gray matter* refers to areas where neuron cell bodies are predominant. The loss of myelin, which occurs in diseases such as multiple sclerosis, causes interference with transmission of impulses.

There are other nerve cells besides neurons, although we seldom refer to them. They are called *glial* cells, or *neuroglia*. They provide support, protection, and nourishment for the neurons and are more numerous than the neurons. Brain tumors are frequently composed of glial cells.

DIVISIONS OF THE NERVOUS SYSTEM

The nervous system can be broken down into subsystems to make it easier to study and understand. These subsystems include the *central nervous system* (CNS), the *peripheral nervous system* (PNS), and the *autonomic nervous system* (ANS). Although anatomically these subdivisions are somewhat distinct, functionally they are interdependent.

Central Nervous System

The two main components of the CNS are the brain and spinal cord. The brain is comprised of the cerebrum, cerebellum, and brainstem.

Cerebrum. The cerebrum is divided into the left and right hemispheres by the longitudinal fissure. Each hemisphere is further divided into lobes with varying functions.

Frontal Lobe. This lobe (see Figure 1.2) plays an important role in personality and complex intellectual functions such as abstract thinking, problem solving, and creativity. The posterior section of this lobe (the motor cortex) controls voluntary movement and houses the motor area for speech (Broca's area).

Parietal Lobe. The parietal lobe contains a sensory area which is adjacent to the motor cortex of the frontal lobe. The sensory cortex receives sensory messages such as pain, pressure, heat and cold, and position of body parts. It is involved in the interpretation of all these sensations.

Temporal Lobe. Impulses related to hearing, taste, and smell are received in this lobe. It also contains a major speech and language center, Wernicke's area.

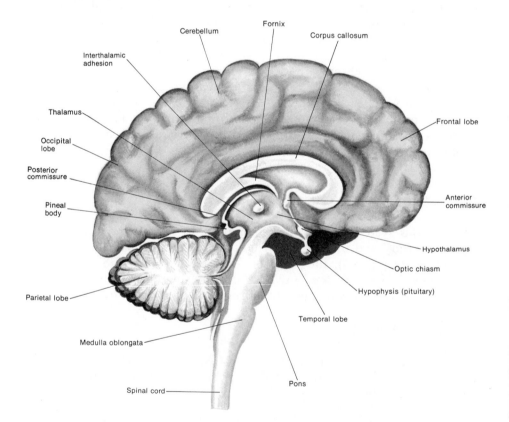

Figure 1.2 Medial aspect of the cerebrum. (From William F. Evans, *Anatomy and Physiology*, 2nd ed., ©1976, p. 155. Reprinted by permission of Prentice-Hall, Inc., Englewood Cliffs, N.J.)

Occipital Lobe.   This lobe, located at the back of the cerebrum, functions in supplying us with vision. Visual messages are sent from the retina of the eye through the optic nerve, optic tracts, and finally to the occipital lobe, where they are interpreted.

Limbic System.   The limbic system is sometimes considered another lobe of the brain, one that cannot be seen from an exterior view. Located within the cerebrum, it is the area surrounding the ventricles. This area is believed to control subconscious emotion and various aspects of memory.

Cerebral Cortex.   The cortex of the cerebral hemispheres has already been mentioned several times. This term refers to the thin outer layer of gray matter of the brain. The majority of the neuronal cell bodies in the nervous system lie in this layer of the brain. It is the cortex that is responsible for initiating all our voluntary actions and thought processes. The functions of the various lobes just discussed originate in this portion of each lobe.

The bulk of the cerebrum is made up of white matter, which lies under the cortex. As discussed, white matter consists of myelinated axons or fibers. Some of these axons connect one lobe to another, some join the hemispheres to each other, and some project down into the brainstem and spinal cord.

Also within the cerebrum, lying deep within the brain, are several other important structures. They include the thalamus, hypothalamus, basal ganglia, internal capsule, and ventricles.

Thalamus.   The thalamus is a relay station for sensory and motor impulses traveling to and from the cortex. All sensory impulses pass through this structure on the way to the cortex. Some motor impulses from the cerebellum and basal ganglia pass through the thalamus on the way to the spinal cord. The thalamus also plays a role in consciousness and alertness.

Hypothalamus.   This is a small but complex structure lying just anterior to the thalamus (see Figure 1.2). It controls body temperature, regulates pituitary hormones, controls appetite, helps maintain wakefulness or sleep, and regulates visceral activities through the autonomic nervous system. The pituitary gland is connected to the hypothalamus and stores some of the hormones produced by the hypothalamus, such as antidiuretic hormone.

Basal Ganglia.   Basal ganglia or basal nuclei are small groups of neuron cell bodies (gray matter) buried deep in the cerebral hemispheres. They are responsible for coordination and smoothness of

muscle activity, especially fine movements of the extremities. Disturbances of the basal ganglia can cause tremors and rigid movement.

Internal Capsule.   The internal capsule is an area that lies between
the thalamus and the basal ganglia in which many nerve tracts from the
cerebrum converge before entering the brainstem.

Ventricles.   The ventricles of the brain are cavities which lie
primarily within the cerebrum. There are four ventricles, called the
lateral ventricles (one and two) and the third and fourth ventricles.
They are filled with *cerebrospinal fluid* (CSF) and serve as shock
absorbers for the brain and spinal cord, absorbing the force of any
impact on the central nervous system.

Cerebrospinal fluid is produced in the ventricles by the *choroid
plexuses*, which are on the surface of small blood vessel groups. The
CSF circulates through the ventricles, into the subarachnoid space
surrounding the brain and spinal cord, and is finally absorbed into the
venous circulation through the arachnoid villi, which are small pouches
in the arachnoid covering of the brain (see Figure 1.3).

Cerebrospinal fluid also serves as a means of diagnosis for nervous
system infections and trauma. It is normally a clear, colorless fluid with
a specific gravity of 1.007. It contains electrolytes, glucose, and protein,
and possibly a few lymphocytes. Normal CSF pressure is 60 to 180 mm
of water pressure if the person is lying down and double that if in the
sitting position. The total amount of CSF for an adult is about 125 mℓ.

Cerebellum.   The cerebellum is located under the occipital lobes of
the cerebrum and is separated from the cerebrum by a fold of the dura
mater called the *tentorium*. Its structure is similar to that of the cerebrum in that it has two hemispheres, a cortex of gray matter, and inner
white matter. The function of the cerebellum is to maintain coordination in movement, posture, and balance, without conscious thought.

Brainstem.   The brainstem connects the cerebrum and cerebellum
to the spinal cord and contains many vital centers as well as insertion
sites for the cranial nerves. Motor nerve tracts from the cerebrum and
cerebellum pass through the brainstem on their way to the spinal cord,
and sensory nerve tracts from the body pass through on the way to the
brain.

Midbrain.   The midbrain (*mesencephalon*) is at the top of the
brainstem, lying directly beneath the *diencephalon* (collective term for
the thalamus and hypothalamus). It is the site of implantation of the
oculomotor (third) and *trochlear* (fourth) cranial nerves and is involved
in visual reflexes.

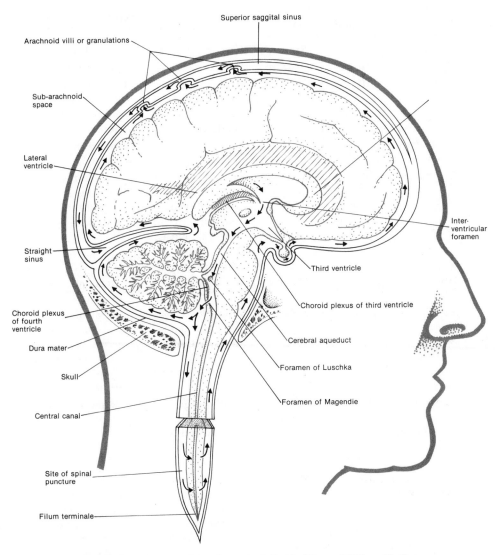

Figure 1.3 Circulation of cerebrospinal fluid. (From William F. Evans, *Anatomy and Physiology*, 2nd ed., ©1976, p. 195. Reprinted by permission of Prentice-Hall, Inc., Englewood Cliffs, N.J.)

Pons. The pons is situated between the midbrain (above) and the medulla (below). The pons contains vital centers for respiration and connections for the following cranial nerves: *trigeminal* (fifth), *abducens* (sixth), *facial* (seventh), and *auditory* (eighth).

Medulla. The medulla is at the bottom of the brainstem where it merges into the spinal cord. Reflex centers for respiration, heart rate,

TABLE 1.1 Important Features of Cranial Nerves

Cranial Nerve	Number	Functional Class	Location of Cells of Origin	Chief Function
Olfactory	I	Sensory	Nasal mucosa	Sense of smell
Optic	II	Sensory	Retina of eye	Visual sense
Oculomotor	III	Motor	Oculomotor nucleus of Edinger-Westphal, both in the midbrain	Eye movements, dilation, and constriction of pupil
Trochlear	IV	Motor	Midbrain (mesencephalon)	Eye movements
Trigeminal	V	Mixed	Trigeminal motor nucleus and main sensory nucleus, both in the pons; also, semilunar (Gasserian) ganglion	Movements of chewing, sensation of the head and face
Abducens	VI	Motor	Nucleus in pons	Lateral movement of eye
Facial	VII	Mixed	Motor fibers: inferior portion of pons; sensory (taste) fibers: geniculate ganglion	Movements of facial muscles, secretion of saliva, taste from anterior 2/3 of tongue
Acoustic	VIII	Sensory	Vestibular ganglion in internal acoustic meatus and spiral ganglion of cochlea	Hearing and equilibrium
Glosso-pharyngeal	IX	Mixed	Sensory neurons (taste): superior and inferior ganglia. Motor neurons: medulla	Secretion of saliva, movements of swallowing, taste from pharnyx and posterior third of tongue, reflexes of breathing and blood pressure
Vagus	X	Mixed	Sensory neurons: jugular and nodose ganglia; motor neurons: dorsal motor nucleus	Movements and sensations of heart, digestive organs, and larynx

TABLE 1.1 Important Features of Cranial Nerves (*Cont.*)

Cranial Nerve	Number	Functional Class	Location of Cells of Origin	Chief Function
Accessory	XI	Motor	Spinal portion: anterior gray horn, upper six segments of spinal cord; cranial portion: nuclei in medulla	Movements of head, shoulder, and voice-producing parts of larynx
Hypoglossal	XII	Motor	Hypoglossal nucleus of medulla	Movements of the tongue

swallowing, coughing, and vomiting are housed in the medulla, making it a vital organ in itself. It is also the point of origin for four cranial nerves: the *glossopharyngeal* (ninth), *vagus* (tenth), *spinal accessory* (eleventh), and *hypoglossal* (twelfth). See Table 1.1 for more information about the cranial nerves.

The brainstem also contains the origins of the *reticular activating system* (RAS), whose neurons are capable of waking and arousing the entire brain. The cell bodies of the RAS are in the lower brainstem, with axons reaching up to the cerebral cortex. When certain sensory stimuli travel up from the body, the RAS alerts the brain, and wakefulness occurs.

Spinal Cord. The spinal cord extends from the medulla down through the vertebral canal to the second lumbar vertebra in adults and to the sacral region in infants. There are 31 segments of the cord: 8 cervical, 12 thoracic, 5 lumbar, 5 sacral, and 1 coccygeal. These segments lie close to but not in exact parallel position to the vertebrae by the same names, since the vertebral column grows faster and becomes longer than the spinal cord.

The outermost layers of spinal cord tissue are white matter; the inner areas are gray matter in the shape of a butterfly. The white matter consists of mostly myelinated axons, which form nerve tracts connecting the brain to the periphery of the body, and vice versa. The ascending tracts (see Figure 1.4) carry sensory impulses from the body up to the cerebral cortex. The descending tracts carry impulses from the brain to the muscles.

The gray matter of the spinal cord contains the cell bodies for spinal nerves. The *anterior horns* of the spinal cord are the lower areas of gray matter, corresponding to the back wings of a butterfly (see

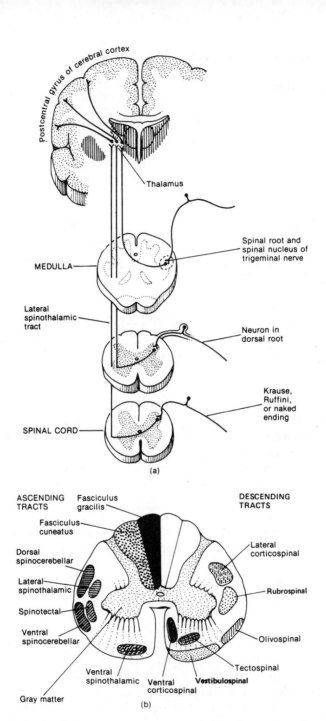

Figure 1.4 Spinal tracts or pathways. (a) A typical three-neuron pathway, the lateral spinothalamic tract, which is the pathway for pain and temperature; (b) location of the major tracts or pathways of the spinal cord. All are bilateral but are shown on only one side of the drawing for clarity. (From William F. Evans, *Anatomy and Physiology*, 2nd ed., ©1976, p. 180. Reprinted by permission of Prentice-Hall, Inc., Englewood Cliffs, N.J.)

Figure 1.4). The cell bodies of motor nerves lie in the anterior horns. The *posterior horns* are the upper gray areas, corresponding to the front wings of a butterfly. The cell bodies of sensory nerves lie in the posterior horns.

In the very center of the spinal cord is the *central canal*. Cerebrospinal fluid flows down from the brain through this canal.

Meninges.   There are three membranes, or meninges, that cover the brain and spinal cord and give it some protection. The outermost layer is called the *dura mater*, the thickest and strongest of the membranes, actually consisting of two separate layers. It lies close against the inside of the skull bones.

The middle membrane is called the *arachnoid mater*. The weblike delicate appearance of this layer gives it its name. There is a potential space between the dura and arachnoid membranes.

The innermost of the meninges, the *pia mater*, is so thin that it is almost transparent. This membrane adheres closely to the surface of the brain and spinal cord. The space between the arachnoid and pia mater is termed the *subarachnoid space*; this is a common site for hemorrhage. The pia mater carries many blood vessels in it, which nourish the cerebrum and spinal cord.

Cerebral and Spinal Circulation.   Arterial circulation to the brain originates from the aortic arch and its branches. Two pairs of arteries, the vertebral and internal carotids, carry blood to the brain tissue (see Figure 1.5).

The *vertebral arteries* supply the posterior portions of the brain: the brainstem, the cerebellum, parts of the diencephalon; and portions of the occipital and temporal lobes. The vertebral arteries merge at the level of the pons to form the *basilar artery*, which then branches out again.

The *internal carotid arteries* provide blood for the anterior portions of the brain: the largest part of the cerebral hemispheres, the basal ganglia, and parts of the diencephalon. The most important branches of the internal carotids are the *anterior* and *middle cerebral arteries*.

The vertebral and internal carotid systems converge around the pituitary gland to form the *circle of Willis*. This anastamosis of the two systems can be helpful in cases of obstruction in one of the branches.

The majority of the arterial blood supply to the spinal cord stems from the vertebral arteries and their branches, the *anterior spinal artery* and two *posterior spinal arteries*. The anterior spinal artery supplies the anterior horns and tracts; the posterior spinal arteries supply the posterior horns and tracts.

Cerebral venous blood returns to the heart by way of veins that

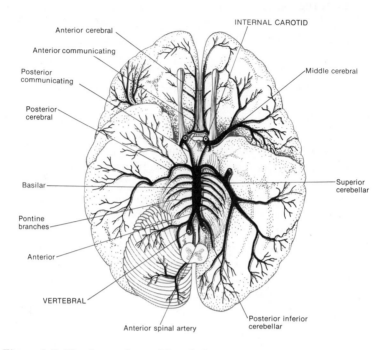

Figure 1.5 The internal carotid and the vertebral artery give origin to the arteries that supply the brain. (From William F. Evans, *Anatomy and Physiology*, 2nd ed., ©1976, p. 198. Reprinted by permission of Prentice-Hall, Inc., Englewood Cliffs, N.J.)

empty into *sinuses*. Sinuses are areas where the layers of dura mater are separated. Venous blood drains through the sinuses and eventually into the jugular veins. Spinal venous blood is returned through the spinal veins that accompany spinal arteries.

Peripheral Nervous System

The peripheral nervous system is comprised of the 12 pairs of cranial nerves, 31 pairs of spinal nerves, and the autonomic nerves. Some of these nerves carry impulses from the central nervous system to the muscles of the body and are therefore called *motor nerves*; others relay impulses from the peripheral receptors back to the CNS and are termed *sensory nerves*. However, many nerves contain both motor and sensory fibers as well as neurons from the autonomic nervous system and are called *mixed nerves*.

Cranial Nerves. The 12 pairs of cranial nerves already discussed are a mixture of motor, sensory, and mixed nerves. They are concerned primarily with regulating and integrating functions of the head, including the special senses. See Table 1.1 for a comparison of the cranial nerves and their functions.

Spinal Nerves.   The spinal nerves exit from the spinal cord at each of the 31 cord segments. The lumbar and sacral nerves have long roots, which fill the spinal canal below the end of the cord itself until exiting between the lower vertebrae. This group of nerves is termed the *cauda equina.*

Each spinal nerve consists of a motor root and a sensory root, which exit from the spinal cord (see Figure 1.6). The motor root

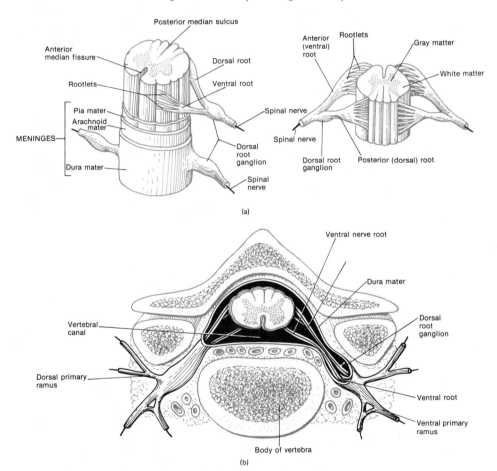

Figure 1.6 A spinal nerve. (a) Formation; (b) relation to structures of the vertebral column. (From William F. Evans, *Anatomy and Physiology*, 2nd ed., ©1976, p. 172. Reprinted by permission of Prentice-Hall, Inc., Englewood Cliffs, N.J.)

originates in the anterior (ventral) horn of the spinal cord, the sensory root in the posterior (dorsal) horn. Once outside of the spinal column, the two roots join to form the spinal nerve. The nerve travels out to the periphery of the body to send out and bring back messages for the CNS.

In addition to nerves that ultimately respond to messages from the brain, there are nerve pathways that function relatively independently of the brain. These pathways are called *simple reflex arcs*. They consist of a receptor in a muscle or skin, an afferent neuron that brings the impulse to the spinal cord, a connecting neuron in the cord, and an efferent neuron that brings the impulse back to the effector (in the muscle or skin). Notice that the impulse does not move up the spinal cord to the brain, so that all action can take place without thought. Reflexes are often protective in nature.

Autonomic Nervous System

The autonomic nervous system (ANS) is an involuntary system that controls much of the unconscious motor activity of the body. It regulates such functions as blood pressure, heart rate, intestinal motility, glandular secretion, sweating, and dilation or constriction of blood vessels. Neurons in this system are located in the brainstem, spinal cord, and periphery of the body, but are ultimately under the control of the cerebral cortex and hypothalamus. The nerve fibers of the ANS travel to the viscera together with the cranial and spinal nerves and the blood vessels.

The two divisions of the ANS are called the sympathetic division and parasympathetic division. The *sympathetic division* is mainly responsible for mobilizing the body's energy during times of physical or emotional stress. The *parasympathetic division* regulates the normal internal functions of the body and tries to conserve energy while doing so. Between the actions of the two systems, a balance is achieved and homeostasis results.

Sympathetic Division. The cell bodies of the sympathetic division lie in the thoracic and lumbar segments of the spinal cord. The axons that leave the cord travel out to the ganglia of the sympathetic trunk. This trunk is a long chain of nerve cell bodies which lies close to each side of the vertebral column (see Figure 1.7). The axons that connect the spinal cord to the sympathetic ganglia are called preganglionic fibers. The preganglionic fibers synapse with second-order neurons either in the sympathetic trunk or in central areas of the body, with the

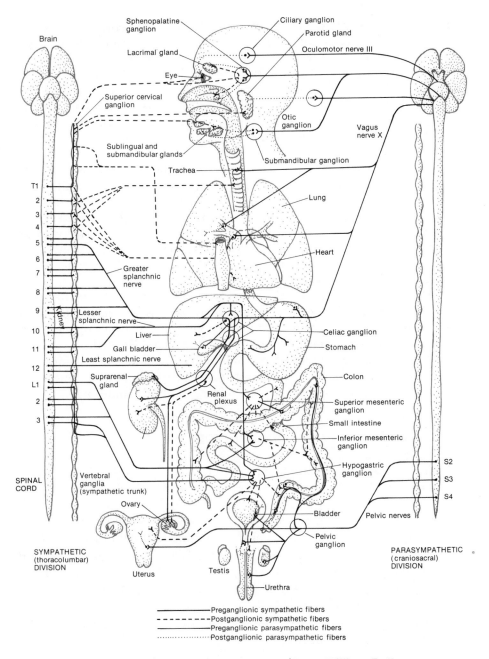

Figure 1.7 The autonomic nervous system. (From William F. Evans, *Anatomy and Physiology*, 2nd ed., ©1976, p. 187. Reprinted by permission of Prentice-Hall, Inc., Englewood Cliffs, N.J.)

impulse carried across the synapse by acetylcholine. The second-order neurons have axons that innervate the various organs, glands, and smooth muscles of the body. The axons of the second neurons are c·lled postganglionic fibers; they release *norepinephrine* and small amounts of *epinephrine* (adrenalin) from the ends of the axons in order to stimulate the various body functions. Because these sympathetic postganglionic fibers release norepinephrine and epinephrine (adrenalin), they are termed *adrenergic* fibers.

Parasympathetic Division. The parasympathetic division has its original cell bodies in the brainstem and cranial nerve nuclei and in the sacral segments of the spinal cord. Axons leaving these areas of the CNS travel out as far as the organs or glands being innervated before synapsing with ganglia of the second-order neurons. Thus, postganglionic fibers in the parasympathetic division are very short. Postganglionic fibers in this division release acetylcholine in order to do their work, and they are called *cholinergic fibers*.

Figure 1.7 illustrates the body's innervation by the autonomic nervous system. You can see that many organs are served by both sympathetic and parasympathetic divisions. The relationship between preganglionic and postganglionic fibers is also demonstrated.

After studying the central, peripheral, and autonomic nervous systems, it becomes clear that they are not separate entities, but interrelated systems that work together to integrate body functions.

REFERENCES

Anthony, Catherine Parker, and Norma Jane Kolthoff, *Textbook of Anatomy and Physiology*. St. Louis: The C. V. Mosby Company, 1975.

Chusid, Joseph G., *Correlative Neuroanatomy and Functional Neurology*, 16th ed. Los Altos, Calif.: Lange Medical Publications, 1976.

Clarke, R., *Manter and Gatz's Essentials of Clinical Neuroanatomy and Neurophysiology*, 5th ed. Philadelphia: F. A. Davis Company, 1975.

Evans, William F., *Anatomy and Physiology*, 2nd ed. Englewood Cliffs, N.J.: Prentice-Hall, Inc., 1976.

Guyton, Arthur C., *Basic Human Physiology*, 2nd ed. Philadelphia: W. B. Saunders Company, 1977.

2

The Nursing Assessment
and Data Base

When you are caring for a patient with neurologic dysfunction, your assessment skills are of the utmost importance. The decisions you make and the interventions you carry out are heavily dependent on your assessments; therefore, they must be accurate, complete, and pertinent to the situation. Before planning care, you must do a baseline comprehensive assessment. After the baseline is established, you can decide which assessments you must continue to make.

This chapter will provide you with information about the data you must look for and ask about, the findings that may result, and what those findings mean. Correct interpretations about the data can only be made if the nurse has a sound knowledge of the significance of certain signs in relation to the functioning of the nervous system.

It is only after the process of assessment has been completed that you should begin to plan individualized patient care. In some cases, especially in respect to the nursing history, there may be an overlap of data collection between the physician and the nurse. If the physician has already completed the medical history, you should consult the history to avoid asking the patient the same information a second time. Patients soon lose confidence in health care providers who do not communicate with each other.

THE NURSING HISTORY

A complete nursing history should be collected on each patient at the time of admission. In this chapter, however, we are concerned only with those portions of the nursing history that have special significance for the neurologic patient.

Find out as much as you can about the current health problem for which the patient is being admitted. It is important to know how long the problem has existed, what symptoms have been noticed, and how they have affected the person's activities of daily living and general life style. You will also need to know about the patient's emotional responses to this illness and how much information the person has about the problem.

For many neurologic patients, baseline information about bowel and bladder habits is valuable, since neurologic dysfunction often affects these systems. Medications that the patient has been taking at home should be investigated because they may have an effect on level of consciousness, coordination, pupil size, or vital signs. Information about allergies is essential, especially medication and food allergies, which may have a bearing on treatment.

Patients who have been involved in an accident and are brought to the emergency department may not be able to provide any information. Instead, ask the family or anyone who witnessed the accident for necessary data. If the patient is now conscious, was there previous loss of consciousness, when did it begin, and how long has it lasted? If the patient is now unconscious, were there any periods of consciousness since the accident? This information may help the physician make determinations about types of brain injury and possible bleeding. Ask if any seizures were noticed and if so, what type they were (see Chapter 9) and how long they lasted. Did the patient vomit since the accident? Was there any obvious loss of muscle function or speech? All of this information can be valuable to the physician in making the medical diagnosis, and will help prepare the nurse for crises that may occur.

Other data that may later prove to be significant are such things as past medical history, family history of neurologic problems, ethnic background, patient's occupation, and whether the patient is right or left handed. Although this part of the history may not have significance in the emergency situation, it may play an important role in planning long-term nursing care that is individualized to meet the patient's needs.

MENTAL STATUS

Level of Consciousness

Level of consciousness may be one of the most important assessments you can make, because the levels reflect brain pathology and metabolic disturbances very quickly, and may be the first sign of a general change in condition.

The terms used to describe levels of consciousness often mean different things to different people, and unless all health care personnel in a facility agree on specific meanings, it is better to describe behaviors rather than to use labels. However, terms are defined in this chapter according to generally accepted usage.

Fully awake.   The patient who is fully awake is at the highest level of consciousness and response to stimuli. A person can be fully awake, however, and still be disoriented or confused.

Alert.   This term refers to being both fully awake and oriented to time and place. Simple questions about the patient's family or job or about present whereabouts elicit correct responses.

Lethargic.   The lethargic patient seems dull and listless, uninterested in surroundings and very sleepy. You can arouse this patient from sleep fairly easily, but when stimulation stops, the patient sleeps again. The lethargic patient can also be either oriented or confused.

Stuporous.   At this level of consciousness, the patient must be subjected to strong stimuli, such as loud voices, pressure on the sternum, or bright lights, in order to elicit any response. The response is usually a purposeful attempt to get rid of the stimulus, rather than a verbal response. Confusion and irritability. also occur. The stuporous patient is sometimes called *semicomatose*.

Comatose.   The patient who has no voluntary response to stimuli, including pain, is called comatose. If the patient does have reflex response to stimuli, such as a gag reflex when the pharynx is touched with an applicator, the coma is moderately deep. If all reflexes are absent, the patient is in deep coma.

If you are unsure of which level the patient is in, just describe the exact behavior and response to stimuli that the patient is exhibiting. Be aware of the fact that there is a difference between consciousness and awareness. The terms just described refer to consciousness (with the exception of *alert*, which refers both to consciousness and awareness). But terms such as confused, oriented, and disoriented, refer to awareness. Consciousness, the degree to which we are awake, is governed by the reticular activating system in the brainstem. Awareness—our ability to understand, think, and feel emotions—is controlled by the cerebral cortex, and is assessed as part of the total mental status.

Degree of Awareness

Assessment of mental status, other than consciousness, includes degree of awareness, memory function, and comprehension of language. You can determine awareness by asking the patient a few questions, such as: "Where are you now?" "What month is it?" "Do you know why you are here?" Correct answers to these questions indicate that the individual is oriented to time and place; incorrect answers indicate disorientation to time and place. *Confusion* is a more general term, referring to a clouding of awareness and lack of clear mental functioning, which may or may not include disorientation to time and place. It is important to realize that a patient may slip in and out of confusion—that it is not always a static state.

Memory function is usually assessed in detail by the physician, but nurses also need to know the memory capabilities of patients they may be teaching. You can test *immediate recall*, a function of the limbic system, by asking the patient to repeat a series of five or six numbers after you have said them. *Recent memory* is assessed by asking such questions as: "What is your doctor's name?" or "What did you eat for breakfast?" This type of memory for recent happenings is primarily a function of the temporal lobe. *Remote memory*, about things in the far past, reflects the workings of the entire cerebral cortex. If you ask the patient "Who was the first U.S. president?" or "When were you born?", you are checking on remote memory.

Language comprehension must be assessed as part of the baseline, to make sure that the patient is capable of understanding you and following directions. Give some simple commands, such as "Stick out your tongue" and "Close your eyes." If the patient does not respond to commands, make sure that poor hearing is not the problem. If it is not, the patient might be confused or have *receptive aphasia* (inability to understand speech). Also assess whether the patient can use language appropriately. The patient who cannot express thoughts correctly may be suffering from *expressive aphasia* (see Chapter 7).

PUPIL RESPONSE

Pupil constriction is controlled by the third cranial nerve, the oculomotor nerve, which originates in the midbrain and is a parasympathetic nerve. Dilation of the pupil is controlled by sympathetic nerves, which also originate in the brainstem. Abnormal dilation or constriction (usually dilation) of the pupils can be due to increased intracranial pressure affecting the midbrain, or entire brainstem, or can be due to brainstem trauma. Constriction or dilation of only one pupil usually indicates pressure on only one side of the brain. Abnormal pupil response can also occur when there is trauma to the eye, such as a direct hit over the eye, or as a result of medication such as atropine or narcotics.

When you assess pupil response, you should be in a darkened

room or at least have the patient facing away from any light source. First, while the patient stares straight ahead, look at both pupils to estimate size and equality. It is a good idea to draw the pupil size on a piece of paper so that you can measure or draw it later on the chart. Do not try to measure the pupils with a ruler near the eyes, because you may cause the pupils to constrict. Both pupils should be of equal size, but up to 20% of healthy people do have slightly unequal pupils. Any large variation between pupils should be reported immediately.

Next, test the pupillary response to light. Cover one eye with your hand while you shine a flashlight at the corner of the opposite eye. The exposed pupil should quickly constrict. Then repeat with the other eye. Finally, shine the light at one eye and watch both pupils. Both should constrict even when only one is exposed to light; this is called a *consensual reaction*. If the pupils show a very slow or sluggish response, you can suspect that complete lack of response (fixed pupils) will eventually follow.

The third assessment you should make about pupils is a test of *accommodation*. If an object is moved up to the face quickly, the lens of the eye changes shape to adjust vision, and at the same time, the iris constricts, causing a constricted pupil. This process is called "accommodation for near vision." You can test this reaction by first having the patient focus on your finger when it is about 12 inches away from the face. Quickly move your finger toward the patient's face while you watch the eyes. By the time you get within 2 inches of the face, the eyes will both have rotated nasally and the pupils will have constricted. This normal response indicates a functioning oculomotor nerve.

Any abnormal pupil response should be reported and recorded in detail. If all responses are normal, the notation "PERLA" can be made, meaning "Pupils are equal and react to light and accommodation."

OPTIC DISC

The average nurse has no need to become proficient at using an ophthalmoscope; this is generally considered a skill of a nurse practitioner. However, nurses working in emergency rooms, intensive care units, and neurological units should at least be able to visualize the optic disc with an ophthalmoscope. The normal optic disc, the point at which the optic nerve enters the retina, is yellowish or very pale pink, has distinct margins, and encompasses a smaller pale yellow area called the *physiologic cup*.

A patient with increased intracranial pressure due to trauma or tumors may develop a sign called *papilledema* or *choked disc*, due to swelling of the optic nerve. In this condition, the disc margins become blurred, the disc is elevated above the retina, the physiologic cup can no longer be seen, and surrounding veins may become engorged. Since the nurse makes more frequent assessments than the physician, it may well be the nurse who first recognizes an abnormal disc and reports it to the physician.

VISION

A complete eye examination, including tests of visual acuity and visual fields, lies within the scope of medicine, and nurses are seldom responsible for more than testing vision with a Snellen chart. But in the case of acutely ill patients, nurses may need to do a gross assessment of vision to determine changes in the patient's condition. The first approach to testing sight is to hold up two or three fingers and ask the patient to tell you how many fingers are seen. You can get some idea of vision if the patient tells you the wrong number or that the fingers are blurred. Diplopia is a possible finding if the patient sees four fingers instead of two.

You can estimate the extent of the visual field if you do a confrontation test, which compares the patient's visual field with your own. While you are facing each other, have the patient close first the right eye while you close your left, then stare at each other's faces. Move your finger along a plane midway between you, starting out where neither of you can see it and gradually moving it into your field of vision. If the patient can see the finger at the same time that you can, the visual fields are approximately equal and normal. Repeat the procedure with the other eye. The normal field of vision is about 50 degrees upward, 70 degrees downward, 60 degrees nasally, and 90 degrees temporally. A restriction in the field is often due to brain tumors or cerebrovascular accidents.

VITAL SIGNS

Temperature

Brain injury that affects the hypothalamus can cause abnormal body temperatures, either hyper- or hypothermia, since the hypothalamus contains our temperature-regulating mechanism. If this control is lost, external medical controls may be needed. Hyperthermia may also be related to pulmonary or urinary infections in patients who are immobile or have urinary catheters.

The various causes of an elevated temperature can be ruled out by careful assessment. Pulmonary infection can be assessed by culturing a sputum specimen and by auscultating the lungs to determine whether there are nonventilated areas or retained secretions. Urinary infection can be assessed by culturing the urine and observing the urine carefully for sediment or cloudiness.

Respiration

A change in the respiratory pattern may be your first signal of a change in the patient's condition, sometimes occurring even before a change in level of consciousness. An abnormal pattern called *Cheyne-Stokes respiration* may occur if there is brainstem or cerebral damage or cerebral anoxia. This pattern is characterized by a period of rapid, and at times, deep respirations followed by a period of apnea (see Figure 2.1), with apneic periods becoming longer as the patient's condition worsens. *Central neurogenic hyperventilation* is a regular pattern of fast, deep respirations that also indicates brainstem involvement. *Ataxic breathing*, a sign of severe injury or worsening condition, is respiration that lacks any pattern or rhythm and may include irregular periods of apnea.

Blood Pressure and Pulse

Neurologic patients may have great variations in blood pressure and pulse, depending on the pathology that exists and premorbid differences. There are a few typical changes, though, that you may see.

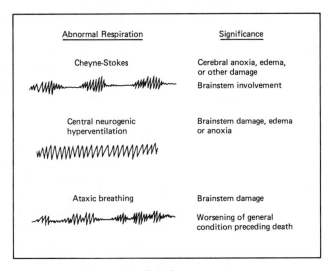

Figure 2.1 Respiratory patterns.

Spinal cord injuries, especially complete transection of the cord, are associated with very low blood pressure and slow pulse. Increased intracranial pressure usually results in elevated blood pressure or widening pulse pressure and bradycardia, although you may not pick up this change until after other signs of increased intracranial pressure have already appeared. The elevated blood pressure is a response to cerebral ischemia due to the pressure on cerebral vessels. The circulatory system begins working harder to try to supply the brain with oxygen.

MOTOR FUNCTION

Assessment of motor function may be done quickly and in abbreviated form in an emergency situation, but must be an in-depth assessment in a stable situation in which plans for all your nursing care depend on the patient's ability to move. You will find that frequent assessments of muscle strength and tone, gait, reflex movements, and abnormal movements are necessary to keep your care plan up to date as the patient's mobility increases or decreases.

Muscle Strength and Tone

The first step in assessing movement is to see if the individual can move all four extremities. The complete absence of purposeful movement on one side of the body is termed *hemiplegia*. The absence of movement in the legs is termed *paraplegia*, and no movement in all four extremities is *quadriplegia*. Many diseases and injuries, however, do not result in complete paralysis, but in partial paralysis or weakness of varying degrees.

To assess upper extremity strength, have the patient first lift both arms and hold them straight out for 30 seconds. Watch for any tendency of one arm to drift downward or waiver more than the other, indicating weakness of shoulder and upper arm muscles. To test muscle tone, flex the elbows while holding the wrists and pay attention to how much resistance you meet. Increased resistance can indicate *spasticity* or *rigidity*; decreased resistance can indicate *flaccidity* (see Chapter 3). Finally, check handgrips by asking the patient to squeeze your hands. Compare the grip on each side; a weaker grip on one side tells you there is *hemiparesis*. Hemiplegia (paralysis) and hemiparesis (weakness) both result from injury to the motor cortex or motor tracts on the opposite side of the brain from the affected extremity, since the motor pathways (pyramidal or corticospinal tracts) cross over in the medulla (see Figure 2.2).

The lower extremities can also be assessed for strength by asking

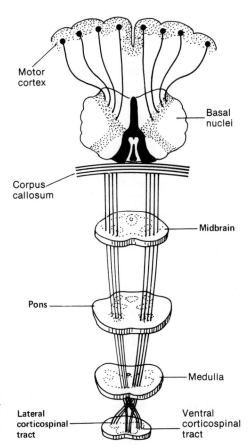

Motor cortex

Basal nuclei

Corpus callosum

Midbrain

Pons

Figure 2.2 The corticospinal tracts. (From William F. Evans, *Anatomy and Physiology*, 2nd ed., © 1976, p. 183. Reprinted by permission of Prentice-Hall, Inc., Englewood Cliffs, N.J.)

Medulla

Lateral corticospinal tract

Ventral corticospinal tract

the patient to lift one leg at a time off the bed. Inability to lift just one leg again alerts you to the presence of hemiplegia or hemiparesis. If one leg cannot be lifted, ask the patient to slide it sideways over the mattress; if there is some weak voluntary movement, the patient may be able to slide but not lift the leg. You should check muscle tone in the legs by flexing the knee as you hold the ankle. The amount of resistance you feel would be described in the same way as for the arms. If increased resistance is felt, try to determine whether it is truly muscular resistance or whether the joints are stiff and perhaps partially contracted. If the resistance is muscular, you should be able to see or feel the muscles tighten and bulge.

Increased muscular resistance can also be termed *hypertonicity*; that is, the muscles have increased tone. If you were quickly to straighten out a spastic or hypertonic limb, muscle spasm would ensue and cause contraction. *Hypotonicity*, which is decreased tone or flaccidity, is easily seen if you lift an extremity and then let it drop. A flaccid limb will drop like a dead weight, with no resistance or muscle contraction. A person can also have normal muscle tone but still have weakness.

Often you can assess gross motor status just by watching the patient's movements in bed or while carrying out activities of daily living. This may be the only means of assessment for a patient who does not understand or respond to commands.

When assessing motor abilities, do not overlook the facial muscles. Observe the eyelids for drooping, called *ptosis*; this condition can be unilateral or bilateral and is due to cranial nerve damage or extreme muscle weakness, such as that seen in myasthenia gravis. Look at the general contours of the face to see if the muscles sag more on one side than the other. Pay special attention to the mouth to see if one side sags or if there is drooling from one corner. Hemiplegia can also involve one half of the face.

Gait

For the patient who is able to walk, you will need to assess the gait pattern. Observe the patient's posture, rhythm, arm swing, and coordination. *Ataxia* is a general term for lack of coordination in walking and may include stumbling, swaying, and staggering. A spastic gait involves stiff extension of the legs and inward rotation of the feet, causing the patient to swing the legs when walking. It is often difficult to determine whether an abnormal gait, especially ataxia, is due to nervous system disease or is due simply to general weakness and immobility.

Coordination

The ability to move in a coordinated, smooth, and even rapid manner comes from the proper functioning of the cerebellum and basal ganglia. There are several simple tests that you should make to assess coordination. First, ask the patient to touch his or her thumb to each of the other fingers, starting with the index finger and going back to it again. Repeat this routine several times, trying to increase the speed. Compare the patient's abilities to your own, realizing that the dominant hand will perform better. People who lack normal coordination will not be able to keep to the proper order or perform the exercise smoothly.

A second simple check of coordination is the finger-to-nose test. Have the patient touch your outstretched finger first, then his or her own nose. After doing this exercise several times with eyes open, have the patient do it with closed eyes. Lack of coordination will be demonstrated by missing your finger or the nose completely or by jerky or tremulous movements. Coordination of the lower extremities is usually assessed by watching the patient's gait.

Reflexes

Reflexes are involuntary movements, some protective in nature, which are responses to stimuli. A reflex movement depends on a functioning reflex arc (see Figure 2.3), which consists of an afferent or sensory nerve connecting the end organ to the brainstem or spinal cord and connecting neurons in the brainstem or spinal cord that link the sensory nerve to the efferent or motor nerve that travels out to supply a muscle. This motor nerve that supplies the muscle is called a *lower motor neuron*. Thus, when a reflex hammer hits a patient's knee, afferent nerve fibers carry the stimulus to the spinal cord. The stimulus is carried across one or more synapses and neurons in the cord, and then to the efferent nerve fibers that supply the thigh muscles, which cause the leg to jerk.

Assessment of the *deep tendon reflexes* (DTRs), such as the quadriceps reflex (knee jerk), Achilles tendon reflex, and biceps reflex, is usually done by the physician or nurse practitioner (see Table 2.1). In each case, the reflex is stimulated by a tap on a tendon, which stretches it and causes the reflex arc to go into action, resulting in muscle contraction and flexion of the knee, ankle, or lower arm,

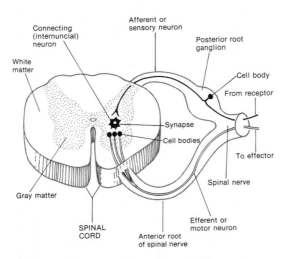

Figure 2.3 A three-neuron reflex arc. (From William F. Evans, *Anatomy and Physiology*, 2nd ed., © 1976, p. 183. Reprinted by permission of Prentice-Hall, Inc., Englewood Cliffs, N.J.)

TABLE 2.1 Reflexes Present Throughout Life

Reflex	Cord Segment Stimulated	Method of Testing	Expected Response
Deep			
Biceps	C5, 6	Firm tap with reflex hammer on:[a] Biceps tendon when forearm is supinated and elbow flexed	Biceps muscle contracts
Brachioradialis	C5, 6	Styloid process of radius when forearm is supinated	Elbow flexes and forearm pronates
Triceps	C6, 7, 8	Triceps tendon above olecranal when elbow is flexed with forearm placed across forearm	Elbow extends
Patellar	L2, 3, 4	Patellar tendon with individual sitting on edge of sitting surface with legs dangling outside	Knee extends
Achilles tendon	S1, 2	Achilles tendon with person in same position as patellar reflex testing	Plantar flexion of the foot
Superficial		With firm pressure, stroke with sharp, but non-traumatizing object such as tongue blade or handle end of reflex hammer:[a]	
Upper abdominal	T7, 8, 9	Upward and outward from the umbilicus	Umbilicus shifts toward point of stimulus
Lower abdominal	T11, 12	Downward and outward from the umbilicus	Umbilicus moves in a downward direction
Cremasteric	T12, L1	Upper inner aspect of the thigh	Testicle on the same side (ipsilateral) of stimulation rises
Plantar	S1, 2	Lateral dorsum of the foot	Toes flex
Gluteal	L4–S3	Gluteal area	Skin contracts in gluteal area

[a]Reflexes are tested bilaterally.

From Esther Levine Brill and Dawn F. Kilts, *Foundations for Nursing* (New York: Appleton-Century-Crofts, © 1980), p. 224.

respectively. Abnormal findings, such as absent, diminished, or hyperactive reflexes, may be related to spinal cord pathology, injury to any part of the reflex arc, or damage to the motor pathways in the central nervous system. Babinski's reflex, which is positive only in babies up to 2 years of age or in adults with pyramidal tract pathology, involves fanning out of the toes when the sole of the foot is firmly stroked. Information about these and other reflexes can be found on the physical examination sheet of the patient's chart.

There are two reflexes that the nurse needs to assess before planning care. One is the blink reflex. If you quickly bring your hand up to the patient's face, you should elicit a blink response, which is a protective mechanism. If it is absent, you will have to protect the eyes from injury or drying. The second is the gag or swallowing reflex. If you cannot see the patient swallowing spontaneously, you should check his reflex. While holding a tongue depressor on the patient's tongue, touch an applicator against the back of the palate or pharynx. The patient should gag or swallow. If not, this patient cannot take food or fluids by mouth and will require suctioning.

Abnormal Movements

There are several abnormal movements that you may see in patients with neurologic problems. Such things as tremors, jerking movements, pill-rolling movements (as if rolling a pill between thumb and forefinger), muscle twitches, and squirming movements are all common and are seen especially in people with extrapyramidal disorders (see Chapter 3).

The unconscious patient may respond to painful stimuli with abnormal movement or positioning. A normal response to painful stimulus is a purposeful attempt to remove the stimulus by pushing it away. A subnormal response would be just random and nonpurposeful arm movements. The comatose patient with severely impaired cerebral function may respond with *decorticate* or *decerebrate* posturing.

Decorticate posturing consists of flexion of the elbows, wrists, and fingers, adduction of the upper arms, rigid extension of the legs, and plantar flexion of the ankles (see Figure 2.4). This posture in response to pain or noxious stimuli reflects damage in the internal capsule or pyramidal tracts above the level of the midbrain. Decerebrate posturing involves rigid extension and adduction of the arms, and extension of the legs, and may be seen when there is little activity above the lower brainstem. Both of these responses indicate that the patient is gravely ill; both may eventually lead to total body flaccidity with no reflexes and a poor prognosis.

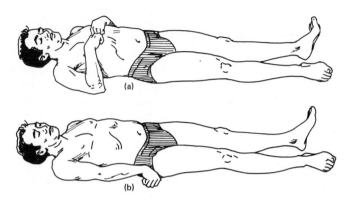

Figure 2.4 (a) Decorticate posturing; (b) decerebrate posturing.

SENSORY FUNCTION

The various types of sensation, such as pain, touch, temperature, and sense of position, are carried by different tracts in the spinal cord and are, therefore, all tested when a complete sensory assessment is done. In-depth evaluation of sensation is usually done by the physician for the purpose of arriving at a medical diagnosis. However, the nurse may do periodic miniassessments to determine any change in sensation that may occur which would affect nursing care.

You can assess the patient's ability to feel pain by lightly touching the sharp and dull ends of a safety pin to various parts of the body while the patient's eyes are closed. The patient should be able to distinguish between the sharp or dull feeling. Temperature sensation can be tested by filling test tubes with hot and cold water, touching them alternately against the patient's skin, and asking which was which.

The sense of touch is easy to assess by brushing the patient's skin with a piece of cotton. With eyes closed, the patient should be able to identify the areas that you touched. You can evaluate position sense (proprioception) by moving the patient's foot or arm in various directions while the eyes are closed. If proprioception is normal, the patient will accurately tell you whether the extremity has been moved up, down, left, or right.

CRANIAL NERVE FUNCTION

A series of simple tests can be performed to evaluate whether the 12 pairs of cranial nerves are functioning properly. Malfunction might be caused by viral infection, trauma, pressure from a tumor, or damage

TABLE 2.2 Cranial Nerve Testing

	Nerve	Test
I.	Olfactory	With eyes closed, patient sniffs nonirritating, identifiable substances, one nostril at a time.
II.	Optic	Test vision with Snellen chart. Check visual fields. Give ophthalmologic exam.
III. IV. VI.	Oculomotor Trochlear Abducens	Tested together. Pupils checked with flashlight for equality, reaction, convergence, and accommodation. Patient asked to rotate eyes in all directions.
V.	Trigeminal	Sensation on face tested by touching with piece of cotton. Corneal reflex checked by touching with wisp of cotton. Patient asked to clench teeth.
VII.	Facial	Taste tested by placing sugar on front of tongue. Patient asked to wrinkle forehead. Observe face for symmetry.
VIII.	Acoustic	Vestibular portion tested by caloric test (ice water instilled in ear should produce nystagmus). Cochlear portion tested with tuning fork (Rinne test and Weber's test).
IX.	Glossopharyngeal	Check gag reflex with applicator against pharynx.
X.	Vagus	Patient can speak with clear voice and swallow normally.
XI.	Spinal accessory	Patient raises shoulders against resistance.
XII.	Hypoglossal	Patient puts out tongue—observe for lateral deviation.

from a stroke. Although the results of the tests may be significant for nursing care, the tests themselves are usually performed by the physician. Table 2.2 gives a brief outline of cranial nerve testing.

ROUTINE ASSESSMENTS

Although a complete and detailed neurologic assessment as just discussed may be done to provide a baseline of information, you also need to develop a routine for making a fast 3- to 5-minute assessment on a patient requiring frequent monitoring. The physician or nurse may order *neuro checks* or *neuro signs* to be done every hour or every 4 hours on a critically ill patient.

TABLE 2.3 Significance of Neuro Signs

Parameter to Assess	Significance
Level of consciousness	Reflects a change in cerebral activity or metabolic functioning of the body
	Often the first signal of a change in condition
	Decreasing consciousness may occur with cerebral edema, anoxia, increasing intracranial pressure, or tentorial herniation
Pupillary activity	Changes in pupil size are due to interference with the oculomotor nerve
	Dilation or constriction of one or both pupils may reveal increased intracranial pressure, brainstem trauma, or trauma to the eye
	Pupil change in conjunction with a decrease in level of consciousness indicates an emergency situation
Strength of hands, arms, or legs	Handgrips are good for quick assessment; comparison of left and right may reveal hemiparesis
	Ability to lift arms or legs is a better indicator of changes in muscle strength; bilateral weakness may be seen with generalized fatigue and muscle weakness or with motor neuron disorders; unilateral weakness may indicate hemiparesis or hemiplegia
Vital signs	Temperature fluctuations may be present if there is damage to the hypothalamus; elevations may indicate infection or inflammation
	Respiratory pattern may be abnormal in brainstem damage; shallow respirations may indicate neuromuscular weakness or cerebral damage
	Blood pressure may be very low in spinal cord injury; elevations and widening pulse pressure may be due to increased intracranial pressure
	Pulse rate may decrease in increased intracranial pressure or increase if general hypoxia has resulted from brainstem trauma

What should you include in such an assessment? It is a good idea to consult with the physician to see whether any specific or unusual assessments should be made. If a nurse has ordered the assessment schedule, the specifics to be included should be written in the card file (Kardex). Individual hospitals may set up standard routines to follow, and all physicians and nurses then know exactly what is meant by *neuro signs* in that institution.

In general, the following assessments are considered neuro signs and are used for quick evaluation of a patient for neurologic condition changes: *level of consciousness, pupillary activity, strength of hand grips* or *ability to move legs,* and *vital signs.* Changes in these parameters can alert you to dangerous changes in condition. The significance of the neuro signs is explained in Table 2.3.

Date and Time	LOC	Response to Stimulus	Pupil Size R L	Pupil Reaction R L	Handgrip R L	Sig.
10/8 10 AM	2	2	O O	/ /	/ 2	E. Smith

RECORDING SYSTEM

LOC	Response to Stimulus	Pupil Size	Handgrips
1= Fully awake and oriented	1= Responds to all commands	Draw size and shape of each pupil	1= Normal strength
2= Fully awake but disoriented	2= Opens eyes to commands, but does not carry them out		2= Weak
3= Lethargic--listless but oriented	3= Responds only to pain or pressure	Pupil Reaction	3= No movement
4= Lethargic and disoriented	4= Responds only with decorticate posturing	1= Reacts briskly to light	
5= Stuporous--difficult to arouse	5= Responds only with decerebrate posturing	2= Sluggish reaction to light	
6= Comatose (unresponsive)	6= No response	3= No reaction	

Figure 2.5 Record of neuro signs.

It is also important to chart your findings accurately and succinctly. Many hospitals have adopted flow sheets for recording of neuro signs, making charting easy and uniform. Anyone looking at the flow sheet can see condition fluctuations at a glance (see Figure 2-5).

ASSESSMENT OF SPECIFIC NEUROLOGIC PROBLEMS

When you have completed your baseline assessment or 5-minute assessment, you will have to make judgments about your findings. Are they significant; do they draw a picture for you; should they lead you to take any action? When you become familiar with signs of some of the important pathological processes seen in neurologic disease and injury, you will be able to decide whether your data warrant immediate action or further observation and data collection. The following are common groups of symptoms that should alert you to possible danger for your patient.

Symptoms of Increased Intracranial Pressure

Since the brain is enclosed in a rigid skull, any significant increase in brain tissue, blood, or cerebrospinal fluid will lead to an increase in pressure within the skull. Intracranial hemorrhage, tumor growth, postoperative edema, or cerebrospinal fluid obstruction may all result in increased intracranial pressure. As the pressure rises, it becomes greater than arterial pressure and the blood supply to the brain diminishes, leading to cellular hypoxia. At this stage, you may see symptoms such as *headache, papilledema,* and *restlessness.*

If the pressure continues to increase, brain tissue is often forced down through the tentorial notch, the only available route. The cerebral hemispheres herniate downward, compressing the diencephalon and midbrain. This tentorial herniation gives rise to further symptoms, caused by compression of nerves and brain tissue. There is *decreased level of consciousness, change in pupil size* (often one dilated pupil), *decreased motor abilities, projectile vomiting, abnormal respiration,* and finally, a *widening pulse pressure.* If unchecked, the process will lead to permanent brain damage and death. It is therefore of crucial importance that you recognize and report these symptoms quickly.

Many critical care units are equipped to do continuous intracranial pressure monitoring on patients with rising or fluctuating pressure. The physician inserts either a catheter or a hollow screw through a small burr hole in the skull into the lateral ventricle or subarachnoid space, respectively. A transducer is then connected to the catheter or screw, and it converts the cerebrospinal fluid pressure to electrical impulses that are visualized on an oscilloscope. Continuous monitoring detects early pressure changes and can prevent crisis situations. The nurse is responsible for monitoring the pressure readings. Rapid fluctuations in pressure can indicate potential danger. High-pressure peaks indicate increased intracranial pressure. Abnormally low pressure may result from tentorial herniation.

Signs of Cerebrospinal Fluid Leakage

After head injury with a possible fractured skull, the patient must be assessed for leaking cerebrospinal fluid. Basilar skull fractures often result in drainage of CSF through the nose (rhinorrhea) or ears (otorrhea). Fluid from either orifice after head injury should be evaluated as possible CSF. Clear drainage can be tested with a glucose test tape; a positive reaction will occur if it is CSF, because of its sugar component. Sanguineous drainage should be inspected as it absorbs into a white tissue or cloth. If CSF is present, the red spot will be surrounded by a clear or bluish wet ring. Report either finding to the physician immediately. CSF leakage indicates that there is direct communication between brain tissue and the outside environment, and a pathway for infection has been opened.

Signs of Meningeal Inflammation

Viruses, bacteria, or blood, when mixed with cerebrospinal fluid, cause irritation and inflammation of the meninges covering the brain. Signs of meningeal irritation are seen in meningitis and subarachnoid hemmorhage, and consist of the following findings. *Headache* is common due to edema and stretching of the meninges. *Nuchal rigidity*, or stiffness of the neck with resistance to passive flexion, is caused by spastic extensor muscles. *Kernig's sign* is often present and is revealed when you flex the patient's thigh. If you then attempt to extend the lower leg, you will meet resistance and the patient will complain of pain. *Brudzinski's sign* also presents itself with meningeal irritation. In this test, if you flex the patient's head on the chest, the legs will also go into flexion. The appearance of any of these signs also requires notification of the physician.

Assessments After Cranial Surgery

Observations that you should make after a craniotomy go beyond routine postoperative observations. You must check the routine things such as airway, vital signs, dressings, fluid balance, and skin color and temperature. But you must also include evaluation of *neuro signs* and assessment of possible seizure activity.

Seizures are always a possibility after surgical trauma to brain tissue. Watch for any muscle twitching in local muscle groups or in the extremities. Also be on the alert for repetitive movements of the fingers or mouth, especially jerky movements. Generalized convulsions can also occur without warning.

Most craniotomy patients develop some cerebral edema, which could progress to increased intracranial pressure. So observe for signs of edema, such as restlessness or slight change in level of consciousness or motor control. Patients will experience headaches from both surgical trauma and edema, but they should not be given analgesics that affect the level of consciousness.

Fluid balance must be assessed very carefully. After craniotomy, especially craniotomy that follows head injury, there is a possibility that the trauma to the pituitary gland will cause reduced secretion of antidiuretic hormone (ADH). The patient then excretes far more urine that is warranted by the fluid intake. Scrupulous measurement and recording of intake and output will reveal this trend very early in the process.

Having completed your assessment of the neurologic patient, you are ready to identify the patient's nursing problems and state them as nursing diagnoses. You can then proceed to planning and carrying out your nursing interventions as they are explained in the following chapters.

REFERENCES

Barber, Janet Miller, and others, *Adult and Child Care, A Client Approach to Nursing*. St. Louis: The C. V. Mosby Company, 1977.

Bolin, Karen, "Assessing the Status of Neurological Patients," *American Journal of Nursing*, 77, no. 9 (September 1977), p. 1478.

Coping with Neurologic Problems Proficiently, Nursing 79 Books. Horsham, Pa.: Intermed Communications, 1979.

Davis, Joan E., and Celestine B. Mason, *Neurologic Critical Care*. New York: Van Nostrand Reinhold Company, 1979.

Jones, Cathy, "Glasgow Coma Scale," *American Journal of Nursing*, 79, no. 9 (September 1979), p. 1551.

Ramirez, Beth, "When You're Faced with a Neuro Patient," *RN*, 42, no. 1 (January 1979), p. 67.

Rudy, Ellen, "Early Omens of Cerebral Disaster," *Nursing 77*, 7, no. 2 (February 1977), p. 59.

Young, Shelley M., "Understanding the Signs of Intracranial Pressure," *Nursing 81*, 11, no. 2 (February 1981), p. 59.

3

Alterations in Movement

The most devastating effects of neurologic dysfunction are, perhaps, effects on body movement, which alter mobility and locomotion and change every aspect of daily living. Whether the damage is in the brain, spinal cord, peripheral nerves, or a combination of sites, the resulting disability can be catastrophic to an individual. The quality of nursing care often determines whether a patient will leave a health care facility in a functioning state or will be incapacitated by complications of immobility and muscle disorders.

PATHOLOGICAL PROBLEMS AFFECTING BODY MOVEMENT

In order to understand the various alterations in movement and nursing modalities used to treat them, the nurse must have some knowledge of pathological processes causing the alterations. The pathological changes covered in this chapter are not an exhaustive list of all the possibilities. The most common dysfunctions and their care are discussed, such as unconsciousness, motor neuron disease, hemiplegia, and paraplegia, with the belief that the nurse must be able to apply basic aspects of care to new but related situations.

Unconsciousness

A patient may be unconscious for many reasons. It may be brief unconsciousness caused by anesthetics or jarring of the brain from a fall, or prolonged unconsciousness as seen in more serious trauma cases, metabolic alterations, or cerebral edema. In all cases, cerebral function is depressed and the reticular activating system may be physically damaged or depressed by chemicals. An unconscious patient has no voluntary control of movement and may or may not have reflexes, depending on the depth of the coma. Nursing care depends, to some extent, on the assessments that have been made about the degree of muscle tone present.

Upper Motor Neuron Disease

All muscles are controlled by two levels of nerve cells. The upper-level cell connects the cerebral cortex to either the brainstem or the anterior horn cells of the spinal cord. These are termed *upper motor neurons*. The lower-level nerve cells connect the brainstem or anterior horn of the spinal cord to the muscle fibers and are called *lower motor neurons*. Thus, any nerve cell whose body is in the motor cortex and whose axon descends vertically through the spinal cord pyramidal (corticospinal) tracts is termed an upper motor neuron (UMN).

Damage to the upper motor neurons may result from a cerebro-vascular accident, brain trauma, brain tumor, demyelination of nerve fibers seen in multiple sclerosis (MS), or by spinal cord trauma, which may crush or sever the descending axons. Whatever the cause, the muscles supplied by the nonfunctioning upper motor neurons are no longer under voluntary control and are therefore paralyzed. They become weak but *hypertonic* or *spastic*. The muscle tone remains because the muscles are still connected to the spinal cord by means of functioning reflex arcs (the lower motor neuron). The *hypertonicity* occurs because the cerebral cortex can no longer exert its normal in-hibitory effects over the reflex arcs, leaving lower motor neuron activity uncontrolled.

Lower Motor Neuron Disease

Any nerve cell whose cell body lies in the brainstem or anterior horn of the spinal cord and whose axons and dendrites reach out to a muscle, is termed a *lower motor neuron* (LMN). Injury to lower motor neurons may result from viral diseases such as poliomyelitis, which attacks the anterior horn cells, or viral-related diseases such as Guillain-Barré syndrome, which damages the spinal cord and causes ascending paralysis. In addition, trauma to the spinal cord will cause lower motor neuron injury at the level of the lesion because of damage to the reflex arcs at that level (the effects of the upper motor neuron damage are seen *below* the level of the lesion). Thus, UMN and LMN dysfunction may exist independently or in combination. Demyelination that occurs in multiple sclerosis and amyotrophic lateral sclerosis (ALS) may attack the lower motor neurons as well as upper, and again a combination of pathologies may be seen.

All lower motor neuron dysfunction results in muscles that are *paralyzed*, *flaccid*, and *hypotonic*, because the reflex arcs have been destroyed, and the muscles are no longer directly connected to the central nervous system. All reflexes disappear and eventually the affected muscles become atrophied. For a comparison of effects in UMN and LMN dysfunction, see Table 3.1.

TABLE 3.1 Comparison of Effects of Upper and Lower Motor Neuron Lesions

UMN	LMN
Loss of voluntary control	Loss of voluntary control
Spastic muscles	Flaccid muscles
Increased muscle tone	Decreased muscle tone
Functioning reflex arcs	No reflex arc activity
Pathological reflexes	No pathological reflexes
Little or no muscle atrophy	Significant muscle atrophy

Hemiplegia and Hemiparesis

Hemiplegia and *hemiparesis* may be due both to UMN problems and to cerebral cortex damage. Brain hemorrhage in the left hemisphere, for example, may damage the primary motor cortex and the upper motor neurons which cross over in the medulla to innervate muscles on the right side of the body. Hemiplegia, therefore, always indicates damage on the contralateral (opposite) side of the brain. By far the most common cause of hemiplegia and hemiparesis is stroke. Stroke is caused by thrombosis, embolism, or hemorrhage affecting a major artery of the brain. The middle cerebral artery is the most commonly affected, and since it provides the majority of blood to the cerebral hemispheres, occlusion of it can have extensive effects on the body. Hemiplegia resulting from occlusion of this artery is typically worse in the face and arm because the motor areas in the brain controlling the face and arm are completely dependent on this blood supply. The leg may suffer only hemiparesis or transient hemiplegia because the area of the motor cortex that controls the leg also receives blood from the anterior cerebral artery. Hemiplegia may be due to damage in the primary area of the cortex, resulting in flaccid paralysis, or can result from UMN damage. In the latter case, muscles of the affected side are still innervated by reflex arcs and usually become hypertonic and spastic after initial cerebral edema and hypoxia subside.

Paraplegia and Quadriplegia

Paraplegia and *quadriplegia* are primarily UMN defects, but can also involve some LMN dysfunction. Both of these conditions can result from either disease (multiple sclerosis, tumors, etc.) or injury (diving accidents, automobile accidents, gunshot wounds). Multiple sclerosis is a demyelinating disease, meaning that the protein and fatty material, myelin, which surrounds many nerve fibers in the brain and spinal cord is destroyed, leaving demyelinated patches which interfere with the conduction of impulses along the nerves. Demyelination may affect only some fibers of the major nerve tracts, resulting in partial paralysis, or can affect all the motor fibers at a certain level of the spinal cord, causing complete paralysis.

Injury can lead to spinal cord compression, partial transection, or complete transection, with partial or complete paralysis. In cervical or thoracic lesions, spasticity will be present *below* the level of the spinal cord lesion and flaccidity will exist in those muscles supplied from the reflex arcs *at* the level of the lesion. With sacral lesions, flaccid paralysis results. The extent of muscle dysfunction (and determination of whether paraplegia or quadriplegia will exist) can be estimated if the cord level of the lesion is known (see Table 3.2). Patients with spinal cord damage, especially with high thoracic or cervical lesions, face

TABLE 3.2 Estimates of Muscle Function in Spinal Cord Dysfunction

Affected Cord Segment	Degree of Body Involvement
C1–4	Paralysis of neck, respiratory muscles (diaphragm and intercostals), and all four extremities. Usually fatal.
C5	Spastic paralysis of trunk, arms, and legs. Some respiratory involvement. Has partial shoulder control.
C6–7	Spastic paralysis of trunk and legs. Has upper arm control and partial lower arm control.
C8	Spastic paralysis of trunk and legs. Hand weakness only.
T1–10	Spastic paralysis of legs and trunk.
T11–12	Spastic paralysis of legs.
L1–S1	Flaccid paralysis of legs.
S2–5	Flaccid paralysis of lower legs but some foot movement. Bowel, bladder, and sexual functions severely affected.

severe disability, including problems of respiration, sensation, and skin breakdown.

Extrapyramidal Disorders

The term *extrapyramidal* refers loosely to those parts of the motor system that are not directly involved with the pyramidal tracts (corticospinal tracts). The extrapyramidal system is comprised of the basal ganglia, certain areas of the cerebral cortex, nuclei of the midbrain and reticular formation, and the cerebellum. Upper motor neurons that pass through these structures are also part of the extrapyramidal system. This system enhances voluntary motor movement by making it smooth, coordinated, and spontaneous. The reason we can climb a flight of stairs without thinking about every step and without stumbling is because the extrapyramidal system is assisting our locomotion. Pathology such as that in Parkinson's disease, Huntington's chorea, and sometimes in cerebral palsy results in the abnormal muscle movements seen in extrapyramidal dysfunction.

The common muscle dysfunctions (dyskinesias) of extrapyramidal disease are disturbances of posture and gait, tremors, uncoordinated jerky movements, and muscle spasticity, or rigidity. The inability to maintain normal or desired body posture results from the failure of the cerebellum and basal ganglia to assess and correct body position in relation to the environment. The staggering, lurching gait typical of cerebellar damage is termed *ataxia*.

Tremors are involuntary movements, which may take the form of constant shaking, often a sign of basal ganglia dysfunction, or shaking that occurs only when the individual reaches out to touch something, called *intention tremor*, a sign of cerebellar disease. *Athethoid* movements are related to tremors, but are slow, squirming-type movements, especially of the face and extremities, caused by alternate contractions of opposing muscle groups, and are frequently seen in cerebral palsy. *Choreiform* movements are more exaggerated jerking, spasmotic motions that may involve the entire body, and are manifested in disturbances such as Huntington's chorea. Muscle rigidity is sometimes seen in disease of the basal ganglia. It is caused by hypertonicity of the muscles and induces a feeling of stiffness and a jerking start-and-stop type of movement, characteristic of Parkinson's disease.

Nursing Interventions

Nursing interventions for alterations of movement must be selected with a knowledge of the patient's particular motor problem. Different modalities are used, for example, for flaccidity versus spasticity or weakness versus complete lack of locomotion. Initial and ongoing assessments of muscle function and functional abilities are the basis for nursing care and rehabilitation.

NURSING MANAGEMENT OF AN UNCONSCIOUS PATIENT

When caring for an unconscious patient, you must undertake all those functions that the patient would normally carry out. This includes all aspects of movement and prevention of complications from lack of movement.

Positioning

You should position a comatose patient in the side-lying or semi-prone position at all times. When a patient is in a deep coma, reflexes are absent, including the gag and swallow reflexes, predisposing the patient to aspiration of secretions and obstruction of the airway by a flaccid tongue. By placing the patient as described above and with the head to the side, secretions can drain from the mouth and the tongue will stay in place. The only exception to this rule of positioning is the unconscious patient who has a cuffed tracheotomy tube or endo-tracheal tube that prevents aspiration of secretions. This patient may be positioned with the head elevated. Also, a 20- to 30-degree head eleva-tion is essential when there is head injury or cerebral hemorrhage. Semi-comatose patients who are able to swallow may be placed in the supine position with the head elevated, or may be lifted into a chair.

Frequent position changes are essential for the unconscious patient. Major position changes (left side to right side) must be made every 2 hours, in conjunction with minor changes (shifting the hips or legs) on the intervening hours. Position changes protect the skin and subcutaneous tissue from ischemia and necrosis, and initiate some movement of respiratory secretions and lung tissue itself, thus prevent-ing atelectasis.

When positioning the patient, take care to prevent joint deformity. Joints should alternately be positioned in flexion and extension, with pillow support to prevent pulling of muscles. If flexor spasticity is present, it is especially important to reposition joints frequently and to encourage extension, thus preventing flexion contractures. The feet should be supported against a footboard to prevent plantar flexion (foot-drop) from the pull of gravity. High-top sneakers can also be used to keep the feet in proper alignment. When in the supine position, external rotation of the hips and legs is a problem and can be controlled by plac-ing trochanter rolls or sandbags on the outside of the hips and thighs.

Your care plan must include nursing orders that are very specific regarding the positioning of the patient. If you want pillows placed a certain way or you find that the patient can only tolerate being turned a limited number of degrees to one side, say so explicitly on your care plan. For example, "Position hip and knee joints in flexion on even hours (pillows under knees). Position same joints in extension on odd hours (no pillows), bed flat." Or, "Position only 30 degrees on affected side for no longer than 1 hour per shift." Evaluate the results of your orders by assessing the patient's joint mobility, circulation, skin condition, and comfort. If your orders were not effective, revise them to meet the patient's needs.

Skin Care

Prevention of skin breakdown requires your constant vigilance and intervention. The unconscious patient, and anyone who is immobilized, is prone to skin problems because of pressure, moisture, shearing forces, and lack of sensation. Changing the patient's position every 2 hours will help to relieve pressure from bony prominences. Although nurses usually think of decubiti in terms of the sacral area, these patients develop breakdown in many areas, including the heels. If possible, keep the heels off of the mattress completely by supporting the lower legs on a pillow. If this is not possible, you can use sheepskin heel protectors.

Skin massage with lotion is helpful in stimulating circulation to a pressure area, but you should not leave the patient with wet skin, since moisture can lead to maceration. Linen should be changed whenever it is damp. Since the shearing force of skin against bedding whenever a patient is pulled up in bed has been found to be a prime cause of decubiti, place the patient on a lift sheet (folded drawsheet), which you can use to bring the patient toward the head of the bed.

Air mattresses, foam pads, flotation pads, and sheepskins have all been successful in preventing skin breakdown, but too often they are not placed on the bed until the skin is already showing signs of pressure. By using these devices from the day of admission, you can avert many skin problems.

Exercise

For the unconscious patient, the aim of exercise is to maintain joint mobility, stimulate reflexes, and encourage circulation. It is impossible to preserve normal muscle tone and size if the patient is unconscious for any length of time. The type of exercise used is called *passive range of motion*. It involves supporting each joint and moving it through its full range of motion at least three times without using force. These exercises should be done twice a day to prevent stiffness or contractures due to shortening of muscles and supporting structures. If stiffness is noted in any joint, you may exercise it more than twice a day, or may suggest a consultation with a physical therapist.

Eye Care

The comatose patient who has no reflexes will need protection for the eyes since the normal protection of the corneal reflex is absent. The eyelids may not close completely, leaving the eyes exposed to injury or drying. Cleanse the eyes with cotton balls moistened with sterile saline every 4 hours, and instill artificial tears (lubricating solution) to prevent drying. Gently massaging the lid periodically over the surface of the eyeball will also help to spread whatever normal tears are present. In addition, the lids may be taped closed with nonallergic tape. Taping is preferable to patching because it is easier to observe the eyelid. It is possible for the eye to open under a loose patch and suffer consequent damage.

NURSING MEASURES THAT MAINTAIN AND RESTORE MOVEMENT AND PREVENT COMPLICATIONS

Patients with neurologic deficits that affect muscle function need nursing assistance to maintain whatever function they have left, as in the case of degenerative problems, or to restore function to the highest possible level, as in the stroke patient.

Interventions for Muscle Spasticity

The primary problems encountered in a patient with spasticity are contracture, pain, and spastic gait. Upper motor neuron lesions produce spasticity. This form of muscle dysfunction will commonly be seen, then, in stroke, spinal cord injury, or cerebral trauma. Cerebellar lesions also produce spasticity, especially noticeable in the patient's gait. Cerebral palsy and multiple sclerosis are examples in which the victims frequently exhibit a spastic gait due to cerebellar damage. Muscle spasticity may be present in a mild form, consisting of hypertonic muscles in a steady state, or can be very severe, causing periodic terribly painful muscle contractions. Spasms can occur in either flexor or extensor muscles.

Exercise.   Since spasticity predisposes to contracture, exercise is of the utmost importance. Contractures may begin early while the neurologic patient is on bedrest during the acute stage of illness, or can occur later in the rehabilitation process. The most common contractures seen are of the affected arm and hand of a stroke patient, or the ankles and neck of a patient confined to bed, although any joint can be affected.

Range-of-motion exercises are used for this type of patient. Because a patient is capable of some voluntary movement, you should not assume that all joints are being moved adequately. Passive range of motion should especially be given to all paralyzed limbs, within the limits of any pain. Besides range of motion, specific exercises should be done with spastic limbs.

Active-Assistive exercises are those where the patient contracts muscles or moves a limb as much as possible, and the nurse assists either by supporting the limb to eliminate gravity or by continuing to move it farther than the patient was capable of doing. This action will increase range of motion and stretch out tightened tissues.

Resistive exercises may be prescribed by the physician or physical therapist and carried out by the nurse. This involves exercises done actively by the patient against some resistance. For example, the patient will raise the affected arm while you provide some resistance by the weight of a hand on the patient's arm (see Figure 3.1). Resistive exercise strengthens muscles and will improve the individual's ability later to carry out activities of daily living.

Patients need to be taught how to do some of their own exercises, if possible. You can teach hemiplegic patients to exercise the affected arm and fingers with the unaffected side. Self-exercise not only helps to restore muscle function, but increases independence and self-esteem. For many patients, exercises must continue for months or years. So it is essential in such cases to teach the patient, or more often the family, how to do passive exercise or how to assist with active or resistive exercise. In your care plan, write your nursing orders explaining what teaching needs to be done, who to teach, how much material to present

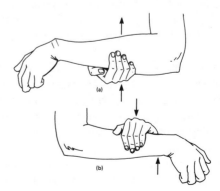

Figure 3.1 (a) Active-assistive exercise; (b) Resistive exercise.

in each session, and how to evaluate learning. Having a family member go through the exercise routine while you are watching is the best way to evaluate whether appropriate learning has taken place.

When exercising spastic limbs, it is of the utmost importance to perform all movements slowly and smoothly. Rapid, jerking movements can trigger severe spasms, which will prevent further movement, cause a great deal of pain, and engender reluctance on the part of the patient to do any further exercising. You will get the best results if exercises are not begun until the patient has limbered up a little in the morning. When nighttime stiffness has loosened up, exercises can be performed with much less discomfort. The limb that is being exercised must be well supported and the rest of the body must be well stabilized, because physical insecurity can also lead to spasms and pain.

Reducing stimuli.   Sudden or unexpected stimuli can trigger muscle spasms in patients with severe spastic problems. Loud noises or sudden movements near the patient can cause painful episodes of spasms. Touching the patient who cannot see you or who is sleeping should also be avoided. Make sure that bath water is not too cold or hot and that the patient is not exposed to sudden cold drafts. Unexpected stimuli cause normal muscles to just contract, but for the severely spastic patient, these stimuli can set off very painful spasms that can take quite a while to subside.

Gait training.   Individuals with a spastic gait, characterized by crossing (scissoring) of the legs, unsteadiness, and foot dragging, can benefit from gait training. This training is done initially by the physical therapist, but follow-up teaching is done by the nurse. The patient will have gone through practice in balancing, in proper weight shifting from one leg to the other, and in proper foot placement. You need to continually evaluate the gait and remind the patient when there are lapses in technique. Sometimes all the patient needs is a reminder to slow down and think about the sequence that has been taught. This kind of follow-up is most effective if you have consulted with the physical therapist to find out precise techniques that the patient is to use.

Positioning.   Just as exercise is needed to prevent deformity, so is proper positioning. Since spasticity often results in flexion of muscles, the extremities should be positioned, for a large part of the time, either in extension or in a functional state. A functional position for the lower extremity is extension with the foot at a 90-degree angle to the leg. No one can walk properly on a leg that is permanently flexed at the hip and knee, and a foot that is plantar flexed. Therefore, when the patient is in bed, most of the time should be spent with the bed flat so that the leg is not flexed. If the patient can tolerate it, the prone position will provide full extension. Periodic flexion is necessary to ensure joint mobility, but this is usually taken care of when the patient is sitting up in the chair, or sitting up in bed for meals. If the patient is on bedrest, you should alternate positioning between flexion and extension.

Patients who experience severe uncontrolled spasms in their legs may not always be able to tolerate complete extension of the legs. They may require a small pillow or folded blanket under the knees. Even this small amount of flexion may relieve the spasticity. Pressure of the feet against a footboard may also trigger extensor spasms in some patients. In these cases, sneakers or heel splints may be more effective.

A functional position for the upper extremity is with the elbow slightly flexed, the hand slightly hyperextended, and the fingers in apposition to the thumb (a grasp position). To maintain this position, place the arm on a pillow, with the hand holding a rolled towel or placed in a molded splint. Plastic splints with Velcro fasteners are made specifically for the individual patient by the physical therapy department (see Figure 3.2). For most patients, the splint is kept on for several hours, then removed for an hour or so, to prevent constriction and pressure on the hand. In extreme spasticity, splints are worn at all times except during exercise and skin care. They are very effective in preventing contractures.

Flexion contractures of the neck can occur if the neck and head are always pushed forward by a large pillow or if the patient always holds the head to one side because of a tracheotomy and attached respiratory equipment. Encourage the patient to move the head from side to side and position the patient without a pillow under the head from time to time.

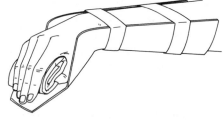

Figure 3.2 Plastic wrist splint with Velcro straps.

Drugs that control spasticity. Muscle relaxant drugs are often necessary to control severe muscle spasticity. When spasms interfere with activities of daily living and with exercise or when they cause pain, relief through drugs is indicated. Diazepam (Valium) has muscle relaxant properties and has been useful in controlling spasticity. Dantrolene (Dantrium) and baclofen (Lioresal) are newer drugs that are also very effective but have more side effects. All these medications can cause drowsiness.

Interventions for Muscle Flaccidity

The patient with long-term muscle flaccidity faces problems of muscle atrophy, edema of the extremities, and joint instability. Flaccidity is seen in lower motor neuron dysfunction such as poliomyelitis or Guillain-Barré syndrome, and is, at least for a short period of time, present in stroke and spinal cord injury. Stroke pathology involves not only upper motor neuron damage, but also some damage to the primary motor area in the cortex of the brain, which leads to flaccidity. This dysfunction is usually temporary, due to hypoxia and edema, and when it subsides, flaccidity also subsides and is replaced by upper motor neuron spasticity. However, in severe cortical damage, flaccidity can be a permanent problem. The person with spinal cord injury suffers from flaccidity during the period of spinal shock, which lasts for weeks or months after the injury. During this time, all reflexes are absent and all muscles below the lesion remain flaccid.

Exercise. Flaccid extremities must be given passive range-of-motion exercise—passive because the muscles are paralyzed and the patient cannot move them voluntarily or by reflex. Although no amount of passive exercise will rebuild muscle size in a muscle that is beginning to atrophy due to lack of innervation, at least joint mobility can be preserved. Atrophy that is due entirely to disuse can be prevented or corrected to some degree by passive muscle contraction. Should reflexes return at a later time, the muscles should be in their best possible condition so that function will return faster.

Range-of-motion exercise also increases circulation. The flaccid limb may become edematous because there is no muscular movement to promote venous flow. Even passive exercise will help to return accumulated fluid back to the general circulation. Edema should not go untreated because it is often uncomfortable and can lead to skin breakdown.

Positioning. A flaccid edematous limb should be well supported and elevated above the level of the heart. Elevation increases venous return and helps to correct the problem of edema. You should assess an edematous limb carefully each day. Measure the circumference of the edematous areas and chart the results. Daily comparisons of size can help you to evaluate whether your interventions are appropriate.

Support and protection of the limb is also important. Flaccid arms or legs easily slide off the bed and hang in a dependent position, subject to damage. If you place pillows to support the limbs and keep side rails up, this can be prevented. If unsupported, a flaccid arm will drag heavily and put great strain on the shoulder joint. The head of the humerus may pull out of the glenoid cavity, a process called *subluxation*. This can be avoided by supporting the arm on a pillow or in a sling. A sling supports not only the shoulder, but also the elbow and wrist. The hand should always be higher than the elbow, to reduce edema.

When lifting the patient out of bed or up in bed, you must use great care. Because the joints are no longer protected by strong muscles, unstable joints could be damaged by pulling on an arm or leg when lifting the patient. All lifting should be done with a lift sheet or hydraulic lift while you support the joints.

Patients who are on bedrest and are being turned every 2 hours should not be positioned on the side of an edematous extremity. You should turn the hemiplegic patient from the back to the unaffected side only. If it is absolutely essential to use the affected side because of skin breakdown, do not leave the patient on that side for more than an hour. Placing the weight of the body over flaccid extremities increases the problem of edema and skin breakdown.

Turning frames.   Spinal cord injuries due to fractured and dislocated cervical vertebrae require immobilization until the fracture stabilizes, to prevent the possibility of even further cord damage. These patients are usually placed in skeletal traction with skull tongs and are to be kept in perfect alignment and immobility. To maintain the proper position and yet prevent complications, patients are often placed on turning frames of some type.

The Stryker frame is very popular because it is easy to handle and is not too frightening for the patient when being turned. With this type of turning frame, the weights attached to the tongs can hang free and maintain traction no matter what position the patient is in. The patient can be either supine or prone, and is sandwiched and strapped between two mattresses when actually being turned. The CircOlectric bed is used to maintain alignment, yet permit turning. The principles of this bed are the same as those of the Stryker frame, but instead of rotation from side to side, the CircOlectric bed rotates electrically from front to back on a circular frame. Although just as safe, patients find it more frightening, especially when turning into the prone position. It is also more likely to cause a feeling of dizziness.

Turning frames make nursing care easier for immobilized patients. Bedpans can be fitted into a hole in the mattress. Exercise and skin care are easier because the mattress is narrow and you can get close to the patient from both sides of the bed. If the patient can move both arms,

self-feeding can be done when in the prone position (the head is supported by straps across the forehead and chin, allowing the rest of
the face free). The patient can also read with a book on a chair beneath
the frame. The patient with skull tongs also requires hygienic care at
the insertion sites. Wash around the pins daily with an antiseptic and
apply a bandage, or coat the area with antiseptic ointment.

A newer type of immobilization for cervical fractures is Halo traction (see Figure 3.3). A steel ring surrounds the head and is attached to
four pins that enter the skull. The head ring is fastened to a plaster
body cast or metal frame, which fits on the chest. The Halo device
allows for earlier mobilization because traction is always maintained by
the device, without the use of weights. Exercise can be carried out with
ease, whether the muscles are still flaccid from shock, or whether
spasticity has begun. The patient can be turned in bed by the use of
turning sheets.

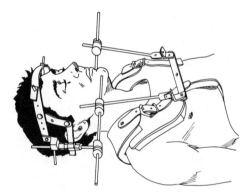

Figure 3.3 Halo traction.

Interventions That Help Control Tremors and Other Dyskinesias

Parkinson's disease, multiple sclerosis, and cerebellar tumors are
pathological problems likely to cause tremors and other dyskinesias.
The nursing interventions discussed here relate primarily to continuous
and intention tremors, rigidity, and various uncoordinated and jerking-
type movements, all of which interfere with carrying out activities of
daily living.

Muscle control. Better control over the hands can be achieved
when the patient is taught to use the upper arm muscles more than the
distal muscles when reaching for an object. When actually trying to
use the hands for fine movement, more coordination usually results if
the arms are held straight out, without the elbows bent. The arm can
also be stabilized by placing the elbow on a solid surface, moving the

arm only from the elbow to the hand. You can teach the patient all these measures quite easily and you should plan for frequent practice.

Wrist weights. Adding additional weight to the wrists in the form of weighted bracelets or cuffs can reduce tremors. The physical therapist will usually introduce this form of therapy. Weighted ankle bracelets are sometimes used to help control ataxia.

Drug therapy. Propranolol hydrochloride (Inderal), a beta-adrenergic blocking agent, has been used successfully in controlling tremors. Because its primary focus of action is the cardiovascular system, the patient must be monitored carefully, should be taught how to take a pulse, and should report a pulse rate below 60.

Muscular rigidity and the tremors of Parkinson's disease can usually be lessened by the drug Sinemet. This medication is a combination of levodopa and carbidopa. Since one of the pathologies in Parkinson's disease is a deficiency of extrapyramidal dopamine, which inhibits muscle stimulation, and since dopamine cannot be replaced as such because it does not cross the blood-brain barrier, its precursor, levodopa, is given. Carbidopa reduces peripheral use of levodopa so that more of the levodopa will cross into the brain. Amantidine hydrochloride (Symmetrel) is also used in Parkinson's disease to control extrapyramidal symptoms. The exact mode of action of this drug is unknown.

INTERVENTIONS THAT SUPPORT CARDIOVASCULAR TONE IN PATIENTS WITH LIMITED MOVEMENT

Patients who have been on prolonged bedrest suffer from two frequently occurring complications, orthostatic hypotension and thrombophlebitis. Nursing intervention can help to prevent or limit the effects of these conditions.

Orthostatic Hypotension

Even a healthy person who is on bedrest for 24 hours can be affected by orthostatic hypotension, and people who have nervous system damage are affected even more. This phenomenon causes a drop in blood pressure when changing position from lying down to sitting or standing, and is due to loss of vascular tone and failure of the sympathetic nervous system to compensate for the position change by constricting the blood vessels. Normally our systolic blood pressure falls about 5 to 20 mmHg when we stand, but is back to normal within 30 seconds. In the person with poor vascular tone, the systolic pressure may drop significantly more than 20 mmHg and will take considerably longer than 30 seconds to return to normal. The person experiences dizziness and syncope because of deficient brain perfusion and if not supported, may fall.

Leg exercises. The patient who can perform active or active-assistive exercises may benefit from a short period of leg exercises before trying to change from a horizontal to a vertical position. Alternately bending and straightening the knee and lifting the leg off the bed several times, first one leg, then the other, may help to reduce the symptoms of hypotension by encouraging circulation and increasing vascular tone.

Support hose. Elastic stockings or Ace bandages on the lower legs will give support to the blood vessels and prevent pooling of blood in the lower extremities. If you apply them while the patient is still in the recumbent position, they also can help to reduce the effects of orthostatic hypotension.

Gradual position change. The paraplegic patient who cannot do active leg exercises, and who may have been immobile for several weeks, should be raised to a sitting position gradually. Orthostatic hypotension in these patients may be extreme because reflex arcs that control vasoconstriction have been destroyed. Position changes may be done first by placing pillows behind the back, and then putting the bed into gradually increasing stages of reverse Trendelenburg position over a period of a few days.

Another good alternative is the tilt table, which can also be gradually raised over a span of days until the body adjusts to the upright position. Take blood pressure readings whenever the angle of the table is changed, to make sure that the cardiovascular system is beginning to compensate.

Thrombophlebitis

The second major cardiovascular threat in immobilized patients is thrombophlebitis, or inflammation of the veins leading to clot formation in the legs. Thrombophlebitis results from pooling of blood in immobile legs and is therefore a preventable condition. It can be prevented by passive or active exercise of the legs, which forces blood in the veins back to the heart, or by the application of support hose, which prevent pooling of blood by externally constricting the superficial blood vessels. In addition to carrying out these measures, assess daily for signs of phlebitis, such as redness, swelling, or pain anywhere in the legs, or a positive Homans' sign (pain in the calf when the foot is dorsiflexed).

INTERVENTIONS TO RESTORE LOCOMOTION

Preparing a patient who has been immobilized or paralyzed for locomotion is a team effort of the physician, physical therapist, and nurse. Weakness, paralysis, spasticity, and loss of sensation can all impair locomotion. Before a person can sit in a wheelchair or relearn how to walk, a good sense of balance must be established. Balance practice is done primarily in physical therapy, but is reinforced by the nurse. The patient practices first sitting balance and then standing, if possible. The therapist or nurse tells the patient when or how to straighten up until the patient recognizes the erect position, or the patient may practice in front of a mirror. By repeated practice, the patient learns how much to lean or not lean and which muscles to contract to maintain an upright posture.

The arm muscles must also be readied to assume extra work in the job of locomotion. Whether the patient is using a trapeze in bed or crutches or a wheelchair, strong arm muscles are essential to aid the body in movement. The physical therapist will first begin a muscle-strengthening program for the upper extremities, and you should expect the patient to practice and to use what has been learned, encouraging independence rather than doing everything for the patient.

Aids to Walking

Braces. The highest goal for locomotion is walking. This may be possible with the aid of braces, crutches, a cane, or a walker. Braces may be of the short-leg or long-leg type, fitting to below or above the knee. Many hemiplegic patients require a brace below the knee to control the ankle, whereas most paraplegics require long braces that also support the knees. You must become familiar with the patient's particular type of brace and learn how to fit it on. The brace is fastened to the patient's shoe and fits around the leg with Velcro straps. A long-leg brace has a knee hinge and lock that enables the patient to sit. Check the skin when the brace is removed to make sure that the metal or straps have not caused any pressure areas.

Many disabled people are able to walk with braces but prefer to use a wheelchair because it is easier and provides faster locomotion. Although a wheelchair may be more practical at times, some walking should be encouraged for the physical benefits of the exercise. Weight bearing on the legs prevents bone demineralization and builds muscles.

Crutches. With or without the aid of braces, many patients learn to walk with crutches or a cane. Crutches may be of the traditional underarm type usually made of wood, or the metal forearm type with a cuff that fits below the elbow. With both varieties, weight is born on the hands, not the axilla or elbows. Crutch tips should be checked frequently to make sure they have not worn through or cracked. A crutch without a good rubber tip to grip the floor is a safety hazard. Crutches can provide stability for the patient whose balance or weight-bearing abilities have been affected. The physical therapist adjusts the crutches to the patient's height and teaches various gaits or walking patterns. You should observe the patient's ambulation for any safety hazards or poor practices, such as placing the crutches too far ahead or too far out to the side of the body, leaning too far forward, or bearing weight on the axilla.

Canes. A cane is useful in providing stability and support if only one leg is disabled. The cane is held in the hand opposite the affected leg; weight is placed on the cane as the person lifts and swings the affected leg. Canes also should have good crutch tips on them. A traditional cane (see Figure 3.4) has only one pole with one crutch tip, but newer types of canes have one main pole which branches into three or four small legs at the base, each with a crutch tip. These are tripod or quad canes, respectively, and are used to give greater stability, balance, and control.

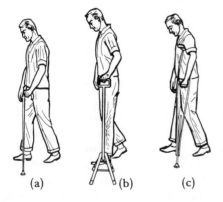

Figure 3.4 (a) Traditional cane; (b) Quad cane; (c) Crutch. (Reprinted by permission; © American Heart Association.)

Walkers. Walkers are usually prescribed for young children or older adults who need a lot of support when ambulating but who cannot manage to control crutches. The person must have enough strength to lift the walker off the floor and set it down about 6 inches ahead. Then, while holding on with both hands and putting weight on the walker, the person walks into the walker. Make sure that the patient is not placing the walker too far ahead, as this can cause overreaching, reducing stability.

Wheelchairs

Patients who cannot walk at all, or who cannot walk without assistance and a great deal of effort, may need to use a wheelchair for locomotion. Wheelchairs come in various sizes with a selection of optional equipment that may make transfers or activities of daily living easier.

Anyone who is confined to a wheelchair for most of the day is prone to pressure areas and skin breakdown. Make sure that there is a 2-inch foam cushion covering the seat of the wheelchair to ease the pressure. Also, the patient should either be repositioned slightly in the chair every hour or should do push-ups with the hands on the arms of the wheelchair every half hour. A nursing order, "Remind patient to do push-ups in the chair Q½H" will remind every nurse of its importance.

Several methods for propelling the chair are available. A manual chair must be pushed by the nurse, or the patient must spin the wheels, usually with both hands. It is possible for a hemiplegic patient to turn the wheel with one hand and guide the direction of the chair with one foot. Quadriplegic patients with high cervical injuries who cannot successfully manage a manual chair use a chair with electric controls, either a pushbutton or the stick type, which responds to light finger or chin pressure.

Transfers. Moving your body from one surface to another is termed a *transfer*. Patients in wheelchairs must transfer at least from bed to chair and back and from chair to toilet and back. Perhaps they may later learn wheelchair-to-automobile transfer. Initially, all transfers are done with the assistance of a nurse, but it is possible for many patients to achieve independent transfers. The technique used depends on the type of disability, for example, whether someone is hemiplegic or paraplegic. Quadriplegic patients with high cervical lesions are lifted in most cases since their arm weakness does not permit them to support their own weight. The basic rules that must be followed in all transfers are that the two surfaces should be about the same height, they should be as tight together as possible, and they should be stabilized.

Hemiplegic Transfer. A bed-to-wheelchair transfer for a hemiplegic patient with the assistance of one nurse is accomplished in the following manner (also see Figure 3.5). The bed is elevated to high

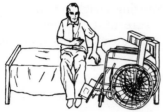

1. Place wheelchair at slight angle to bed, on patient's strong side, facing foot of bed. Keep the right front corner of the chair as close to the bed as possible as shown below.* Brakes locked. Footrests up.

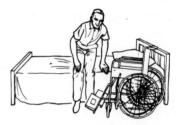

2. Keep feet beneath body, lean forward placing strong hand near edge of bed and push to standing position keeping weight well over strong foot.

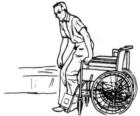

3. When standing position is steady enough for momentary release of support by strong hand, move strong hand to farther arm rest of wheelchair. Keeping body weight well forward, turn on strong foot and lower to sitting position.

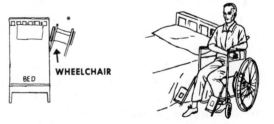

Figure 3.5 Moving into a wheelchair from bed. *Note*: An armchair can be used by the bed instead of a wheelchair. A chair that is heavy enough not to slide and with a firm seat that is not too soft or too low will be suitable. (Reprinted by permission; © American Heart Association.)

Fowler's position. The wheelchair should be next to the bed on the patient's *unaffected* side, the back of the chair about even with the back of the mattress, and the brakes locked. For the safest transfer, the patient should wear a belt around the waist that you can hold firmly. The patient is assisted to a dangling position on the side of the bed and remains there until stable and balanced. You face the patient, both hands on the waist belt and one knee against the patient's affected knee. As the patient attempts to stand, assist by pulling a little on the belt. Most of the patient's weight should be on the unaffected leg while you push against the affected knee to stabilize it. The patient then reaches for the farthest side of the wheelchair with the unaffected hand while pivoting on the unaffected leg. Teach the patient not to sit until the edge of the seat can be felt against the back of the legs.

Transferring from the wheelchair to the bed necessitates using *the other side of the bed* so that the bed is again on the patient's unaffected side. The same basic procedure is then followed. When the patient is ready to move from the dangling position on the side of the bed back into the bed, the unaffected leg is placed under the affected leg, lifting it up on to the mattress as the patient lies back and rolls slightly to the unaffected side. As the patient gains strength, the same regimen can be followed independently. It can also be adapted slightly for a wheelchair-to-toilet transfer if there is a raised toilet seat and a handrail on the unaffected side (see Figure 3.6).

Paraplegic Transfer. Although the paraplegic patient is hampered by two paralyzed legs, there is a great advantage in having two functioning arms, which can be strengthened until they can hold all of the body weight. A bed-to-wheelchair transfer for this patient can be done several ways; the two most popular methods will be described.

Transfer by means of a sliding board is most appropriate for a patient who cannot use the arms alone to lift and move the body. A wheelchair with removable armrests is required. The chair is placed parallel to the bed with the armrest next to the bed removed and the brakes locked. The patient sits up and then dangles on the side of the bed. At first, the patient may need you to support the legs and help place the sliding board, but independence is achieved quickly. The sliding board is placed with one end on the bed and one on the chair seat. The patient rotates slightly so that the hips are toward the chair and the knees are away from it (pointed toward the foot of the bed). By raising the buttocks, one end of the sliding board can be slipped under the body, and the arms are then used to slide the body across the board and into the chair. The patient raises the other buttock to pull the board out, and the armrest can be replaced.

The second transfer method, sometimes called an anterior-posterior

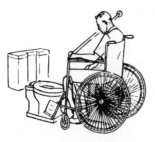

1. Position wheelchair facing the toilet. Brakes on, footrests up.

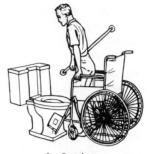

2. Stand up

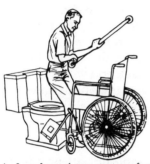

4. Lean forward, turn on strong foot and slowly sit down on toilet seat.

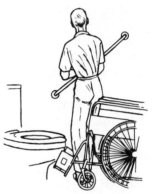

3. Place strong hand on wall bar (or on far side of toilet seat if no wall bar is present).

Figure 3.6 Moving from a wheelchair to toilet. *Note*: Wall bar can be used for support. The patient can be taught to unfasten his trousers before getting out of the wheelchair so that they fall when he stands. A female patient can stand in front of commode instead of sitting down immediately and either lean against the wall or push her strong leg against the commode for support to free her strong hand to handle her clothing. (Reprinted by permission; © American Heart Association.)

transfer, is done with the wheelchair placed so that the seat faces the bed, with the footrests swung outward. The patient must have good balance and be able to lift and slide the entire body with the arms. The patient sits up in bed and turns sideways with the legs across the bed and the back to the wheelchair seat (see Figure 3.7). The arms can then grasp the armrests and push the body up and back completely into the chair. The chair is unlocked and backed away from the bed so that the legs can be lowered onto the footrests. Both of these methods can be reversed to transfer from the wheelchair back to the bed.

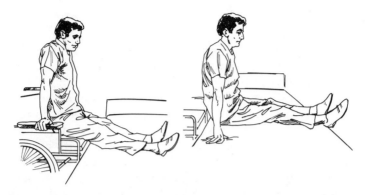

Figure 3.7 Vertical transfer of a paraplegic patient. The wheelchair is placed facing the bed with the wheels locked and the pedals in the "down" position. The patient pushes up on his hands and arms and slides his body forward onto the bed. This is a non-weight-bearing transfer in which the patient is able to transfer on the same level. With conditioning and practice, this transfer can be done to a higher or lower level by the push-up method. (From Lillian Sholtin Brunner, and Doris Smith Suddarth, *Textbook of Medical-Surgical Nursing*, 4th ed., 1980. Reprinted by permission of J. B. Lippincott Company.)

All these nursing measures to promote ambulation and locomotion need to be adapted somewhat to the individual patient. You must evaluate your interventions to see if they are successful for this patient, and if not, plan to find a better way. Ongoing assessment, planning, and evaluation are essential to meet the individual's needs and to adapt to changes in the patient's condition.

NURSING MEASURES THAT HELP THE DISABLED PATIENT PERFORM ACTIVITIES OF DAILY LIVING

Patients with impaired movement may be able to perform various activities of daily living independently, depending on their particular pathology and the modification of approaches to fit their capabilities. The paraplegic person is most able to carry out activities of daily living since the majority of those activities can be performed if both arms are functional and strong. The hemiplegic patient (unless very elderly or debilitated) can be taught most activities if adaptive devices are used. The quadriplegic with a low cervical lesion (C7–8) can manage quite well with adaptive devices, but with a high cervical lesion (C5–6), only limited self-care can be expected.

Hygiene

One of the activities most important to an individual is personal hygiene. The hemiplegic patient who is capable of learning can be trained to do many two-handed or bilateral chores with only one hand. If the affected side is the dominant hand, the patient can be retrained to use the nondominant hand. Bathing or showering and mouth care are possible with only a few adaptations. The biggest difficulty in bathing is washing the unaffected arm. This can be done best with a long-handled sponge or brush, and the arm can be dried by rolling and rubbing it on a towel. A tub bath is feasible for a hemiplegic patient in the hospital and at home if transfer technique has been mastered and certain safety precautions are taken. There must be a hand rail next to the bath tub, and there must be a nonskid rubber mat in it.

Brushing the teeth requires stabilizing the brush on a flat surface with the affected hand or a holder while squeezing the toothpaste with the good hand. The affected hand can be used very effectively in this way to stabilize or hold objects, even if it cannot be used for fine control. Brushing dentures may require a brush fastened to the sink with suction cups over which the patient can rub the dentures, or dentures may be soaked.

Hair grooming can be managed with one hand if the hairstyle is fairly simple. You will have to assist with shampoos or setting a woman's

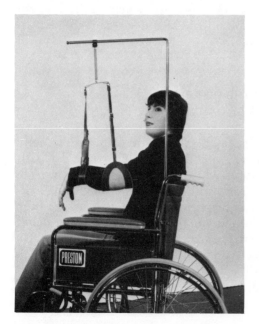

Figure 3.8 Arm sling support for a quadriplegic patient. (Reprinted by permission; © J. A. Preston Corp., 1981.)

hair if necessary. A male patient can shave with an electric razor, although he may need help to clean the razor.

You must encourage self-care as the patient improves, and not be tempted to do everything for the patient just because it will get done faster. Becoming independent in daily hygiene is a milestone for the hemiplegic patient and is a great boost for self-esteem. On the other hand, you should not allow a patient to struggle with a task to the point of complete frustration without offering some help. Encourage the patient to use the affected arm and hand as much as possible, even though movement and control may be limited.

The quadriplegic patient may be able to do at least light bathing and mouth care with the help of arm supports attached to the wheelchair (see Figure 3.8), which suspend the arm and enable considerable movement. If there is no finger control, a hand strap with a clasp on it can be worn to clasp a toothbrush or other small implements. Paraplegic and quadriplegic patients can also shower if they can transfer to a shower chair or tub seat (see Figure 3.9) or be lifted by a hydraulic lift. A quadriplegic patient will need some assistance with showering, however.

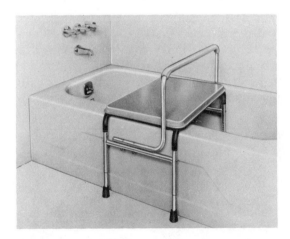

Figure 3.9 Tub seat. (Reprinted by permission; © J. A. Preston Corp., 1981.)

Eating

All patients with weak or paralyzed upper extremities or with severe tremors will need some assistance with eating. At first you must cut the meat, open containers, and so on, but gradually the patient, especially the hemiplegic, may learn to do some of this independently.

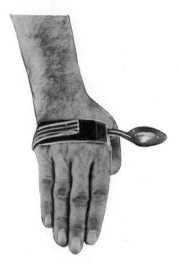

Figure 3.10 Hand strap used to hold utensils or other small implements. (Reprinted by permission; © J. A. Preston Corp., 1981.)

Warn the patient against trying to eat large uncut pieces of meat, which can obstruct the throat. A knife with a curved blade can be used to cut meat by rocking it back and forth.

Utensils with fat handles are easiest to manage. You can pad a regular utensil handle with rubber tubing to make it larger. If the hands tremble, weighted utensils may make the hands steadier. A hand strap with a clasp (see Figure 3.10) may enable patients with weak fingers to hold a utensil. A detachable plate rim (see Figure 3.11) can be fitted onto a plate to prevent food from being pushed off the edge while it is being manipulated onto the fork.

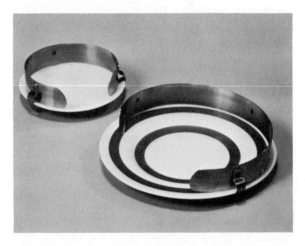

Figure 3.11 Detachable plate rim. (Reprinted by permission; © J. A. Preston Corp., 1981.)

Some means must be found to make mealtimes a pleasurable, non-frustrating experience, or the patient's nutritional status will suffer. Too often, disabled patients eat a few bites and give up rather than ask for help, and too often nurses just remove a tray without finding out why the patient did not eat.

Dressing

In an acute care facility, patients will generally wear only pajamas and robes, but if they learn how to don these clothes, they will later be able to apply the same principles to street clothes. They should practice

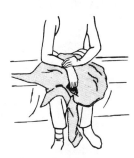

1. Spread shirt on lap inside up and collar away from body.

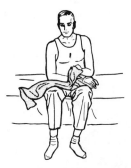

2. Using strong hand place weak hand in right armhole and pull sleeve up weak arm.

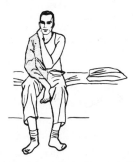

3. Throw the rest of the garment behind the body and pull right sleeve all the way up.

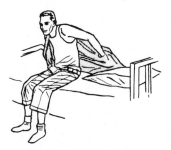

4. Reach behind with strong hand, and place it in left armhole. Work sleeve into position.

Figure 3.12 Putting on a shirt or dress. *Note*: Dressing while sitting on side of bed is easier than in wheelchair if balance is good. IF BALANCE IS POOR, HAVE PATIENT SIT IN WHEELCHAIR OR HEAVY ARM-CHAIR TO DRESS. An open-down-the-front dress, sweater or coat is put on the same way as a shirt but it is necessary to stand up and straighten the skirt before it can be fastened. Large buttons are easier to fasten than snaps. (Reprinted by permission; © American Heart Association.)

with various types of garments and fasteners to find out which they can manage. Practice in dressing can begin when the patient has achieved sitting balance.

The hemiplegic patient should always follow the procedure of putting the affected extremity into the garment before the unaffected one, and should reverse the process when removing the garment, removing the unaffected extremity first. You will follow the same routine when dressing a hemiplegic patient. A shirt or blouse is put on by placing it over the affected hand and sliding it as far up the arm as possible. The unaffected hand can reach behind the neck and grasp the collar of the garment, pulling it across the back, and the unaffected arm can then slide into the free sleeve (see Figure 3.12). Some patients may be able to manage buttons, but Velcro closures are definitely the easiest.

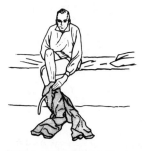

1. Sitting on side of bed, with strong hand cross weak leg, pull right pants leg over weak foot.

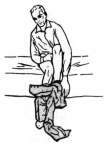

2. Place strong foot in left pants leg and pull pants up as far as possible.
   • If patient cannot stand without support, lie down and proceed as illustrated in steps 3 and 4.
   • If patient can stand without support, proceed to step 2a.

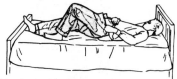

3. Lie down; bend strong knee and hip pushing strong foot against bed to raise hips. Pull pants up over hips.

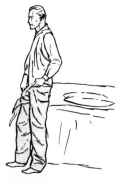

2a. If standing balance against bed without support of strong hand is possible, stand leaning against bed for support and pull up pants with strong hand.

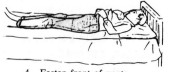

4. Fasten front of pants.

Figure 3.13 Putting on trousers. (Reprinted by permission; © American Heart Association.)

Pants are put on by first placing the affected leg in one pants leg, then the unaffected leg, and gradually pulling them up over the hips. This can be done while sitting on the side of the bed if the patient can stand to pull the pants over the hips (see Figure 3.13). For weaker patients, dressing is easier and safer if done in bed. Paraplegic patients also put pants on while lying in bed since they can roll from side to side until the pants can be pulled up over each hip.

A general rule to follow in selecting clothes is that they should be loose enough to put on without a struggle and should be suitable for adaptation to any devices used. For example, crutch users are more comfortable if armholes are loose enough to allow free arm and shoulder movement, and for brace wearers, pants legs must be wide enough to fit loosely over braces. Shoes should allow for possible foot edema. Tie shoes are usually the best, and can be tied in a way that can be managed with one hand (see Figure 3.14). If there is no swelling, slip-on shoes are easiest to manage. Quadriplegics, or any patient with weak upper extremities, may need continued help with dressing, especially with fasteners.

Role of Occupational Therapists

The role of the occupational therapist varies widely among institutions, but generally it involves retraining of the upper extremities to regain useful function for daily living and vocational pursuits. Sometimes these therapists are involved in retraining for activities of daily living, and will be responsible for the teaching plan. If this is the case,

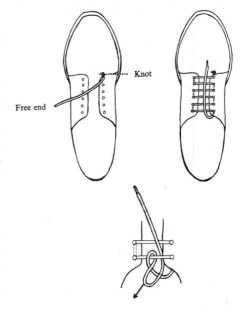

Figure 3.14 Tying a shoe one-handed. 1. Knot one end of the shoe string and lace the shoe leaving the knotted end at the lowest eyelet. 2. In the top eyelet feed the end of the shoe string from outside to inside and throw the end over the top of the laces. 3. Make a loop in the free end of the shoe lace and pull it loop within a loop as shown in 2. 4. Pull the lace tight being careful not to pull the free end all the way through. 5. To untie, pull the free end. *Note*: Elastic shoelaces are available but are not preferred if patient can tie laces. The above type of shoes are preferable to loafers. (Reprinted by permission; © American Heart Association.

there must be good communication between the occupational therapist and the nurse, so that you can follow through with the same
approaches which are used in occupational therapy.

LONG-TERM REHABILITATION

When the disabled patient is discharged from the acute care or rehabilitation facility, rehabilitation does not stop. Most patients still return to
the facility on an outpatient basis for physical, occupational, or vocational therapy or to various clinics for evaluation, or they have nurses
or therapists visiting in their homes. Functional return after neurologic
damage may continue for a few years, in some cases necessitating continuing therapy.

Discharge Planning

The nurse, social worker, therapists, physician, patient, and family
work together when making plans for a patient's return to the community. Most important is the issue of where and with whom the patient
will live. If the place of residence must change, drastic adjustments may
again be asked of the patient. Alterations may also have to be made in
the residence. If the patient uses a wheelchair, ramps or elevators will
have to be installed. Doorways may have to be widened, furniture re-
arranged, handrails installed, and if the patient is a homemaker, kitchen
cabinets and counters may have to be altered to allow the person to
work while sitting in a wheelchair.

Various adaptive devices may be needed in the home, such as a
raised toilet seat or commode, a trapeze on the bed, an exercise pulley
fitted over a door, or kitchen utensils adapted for one-handed use.

The amount of assistance the patient will need is discussed with
the person or people with whom the patient will live. The nurse and
therapists may have to do a lot of teaching to prepare these people to
assist in care. They may also need a lot of emotional support as they
realize the responsibilities they are taking on. Allowing the patient to
spend a few weekends at home before the time of discharge is a valuable practice that often points up learning needs or practical difficulties
not previously considered.

Community Resources

There are many community agencies and organizations that can
aid the disabled person in the community. The social worker is probably
the best source of knowledge about services available in a particular

area. Linking a patient up with such agencies as the National Easter Seal Society for Crippled Children and Adults, the National Multiple Sclerosis Society, the Division of Vocational Rehabilitation, and Meals-on-Wheels programs may make possible a successful return to the community. Some of these resources provide funding; some provide transportation, recreation, and socialization; some provide home care or meals. You can initiate these contacts independently in some cases, or you can work through the social worker.

Psychosocial Adjustment

Long-term or permanent disability involving motor activities drastically changes a person's life style. As already seen, the disability may interfere with the person's ability to eat, maintain hygiene, walk, or get dressed. It may very well mean a change of residence, change of or loss of occupation, and reduction in social contacts and recreational activities. Disability may cripple self-esteem and feelings of self-worth.

The disabled person cannot usually accept all these changes easily or quickly. Just as physical rehabilitation is a prolonged process, so is emotional and social rehabilitation. Nurses can aid the patient and family in making the needed adjustments, coping with the changes, and finding the support that is needed. Specific approaches that nurses may use are discussed in Chapter 10.

EXAMPLES OF NURSING DIAGNOSES RELATED TO ALTERATIONS IN MOVEMENT[1]

Impaired mobility of left arm and leg related to cerebral pathology; beginning spasticity in both arm and leg.

Impaired mobility related to cerebral trauma; unable to turn or position self.

Impaired mobility of all extremities related to spinal cord injury; complete paralysis of legs; has partial upper arm control.

Alteration in skin integrity related to immobility; unable to turn from side to side.

Potential contractures of right arm and leg joints related to spasticity.

---

[1] Diagnoses can be made more specific in a patient situation where a full assessment of data has been done. These diagnoses and others that you can devise based on your data collection can be used in writing nursing care plans.

Potential for injury to left eye related to inability to close eyelid.

Potential for injury related to ataxia and impaired sense of balance.

Potential for injury due to continuous hand tremors, which are worse during stress.

Lack of knowledge related to proper use of walker.

Anxiety related to difficulty in mastering transfer technique.

Alteration in self-care activities related to overdependence on nurses for hygiene and grooming.

Alteration in self-care activities; inability to feed self related to weakness of arms and hands.

REFERENCES

Adams, Nancy R., "Prolonged Coma: Your Care Makes All the Difference," *Nursing 77*, 7, no. 8 (August 1977), p. 21.

Beland, Irene L., and Joyce Y. Passos, *Clinical Nursing: Pathophysiological and Psychosocial Approaches*, 3rd ed. New York: Macmillan Publishing Co., Inc., 1975.

Birrer, Cynthia, *Multiple Sclerosis: A Personal View*. Springfield, Ill.: Charles C Thomas, Publisher, 1979.

Brower, Phyllis, and Dorothy Hicks, "Maintaining Muscle Function in Patients on Bedrest," *American Journal of Nursing*, 72, no. 7 (July 1972), p. 1250.

Catanzaro, Marci, "Nursing Care of the Person with MS," *American Journal of Nursing*, 80, no. 2 (February 1980), p. 286.

Chusid, Joseph G., *Correlative Neuroanatomy and Functional Neurology*, 16th ed. Los Altos, Calif.: Lange Medical Publications, 1976.

Gordon, Janet, "CircOlectric Beds: Circumventing the Trauma of Positioning," *Nursing*, 77, 7, no. 2 (February 1977), p. 42.

Hawley, Donna, and Diana Whitney Reiser, "Reducing Muscle Spasms in a Child with Cerebral Palsy," *American Journal of Nursing*, 78, no. 7 (July 1978), p. 1214.

Ince, Laurence P., *The Rehabilitation Medicine Services*. Springfield, Ill.: Charles C Thomas, Publisher, 1974.

Larrabee, June Hansen, "The Person with a Spinal Cord Injury: Physical Care during Early Recovery," *American Journal of Nursing*, 77, no. 8 (August 1977), p. 1320.

Macleod, John, ed., *Davidson's Principles and Practices* ، 12th ed. New York: Churchill Livingstone, 1977.

McDonnell, Margaret, and others, "MS—Problem Oriented Nursh. Plans," *American Journal of Nursing*, 80, no. 2 (February 1ᵌ p. 292.

Murray, Ruth, and others, *The Nursing Process in Later Maturity*. Englewood Cliffs, N.J.: Prentice-Hall, Inc., 1980.

O'Brien, Mary T., and Phyllis J. Pallett, *Total Care of the Stroke Patient*. Boston: Little, Brown and Company, 1978.

Stillman, Margot J., "Stroke! Pulling Your Patient through the Acute Stage," *RN*, 42, no. 10 (October 1979), p. 55.

Stillman, Margot J., "Stroke! How to Care for a Recovering Patient," *RN*, 42, no. 11 (November 1979), p. 49.

Sutton, Neville, *Injuries of the Spinal Cord*. London: Butterworth and Co. Ltd., 1973.

Wehrmaker, Suzanne L., and Joann R. Wintermute, *Case Studies in Neurological Nursing*. Boston: Little, Brown and Company, 1978.

4

Alterations in Elimination of Body Wastes

Management of elimination problems is one of the greatest concerns in caring for patients with neurologic dysfunction. The person who has lost excretory control faces drastic changes in self-image, life style, and independence. Rehabilitation to activities of daily living is of little value until some type of excretory control has first been reestablished.

PHYSIOLOGY OF NORMAL VOIDING

Normal Voiding

We normally feel the first urge to void when there is about 200 mℓ of urine in the bladder. This urge can be consciously ignored until the bladder holds about 350 to 400 mℓ. At this point, the collection of urine stretches the bladder walls to the point where reflex arcs at the second to fourth sacral segment of the spinal cord are stimulated. The smooth muscle of the bladder then contracts, which gives rise to the urge to void. So far, this action is under the involuntary control of the autonomic nervous system.

Several areas in the brain also have control over urination. Messages are sent from the brain to the sacral segment of the spinal cord via nerve tracts which either permit or inhibit urination. If physical and environmental conditions permit, the brain sends the signal and the urethral sphincters relax and allow voiding. The brain also causes the bladder to continue with contractions until all urine has been expelled. Voluntary aspects of urination, therefore, are present only if the brain is able to send messages to the sacral segments of the cord. Otherwise, the bladder will empty by reflex and may not empty completely.

PATHOPHYSIOLOGY OF NEUROGENIC BLADDER

The term *neurogenic bladder* refers to dysfunction related to a change in innervation of the bladder, either in the autonomic or central nervous systems, or to cerebral dysfunction. Several types of neurogenic bladder will be discussed, together with the alternatives of nursing management.

Upper Motor Neuron Bladder

There are two causes of neurogenic bladder that affect the upper motor neurons. One cause is cerebral pathology, such as brain tumors, cerebrovascular accidents, or brain injury; the other is upper spinal cord injury (above T12). In both cases, the brain cannot send out the normal messages to the bladder and sphincter which serve to keep voiding under conscious control. Instead, the bladder functions simply by reflex activity because the reflex arcs are still intact. A bladder which functions in this manner is termed an *upper motor neuron bladder* or a *reflex bladder*. The bladder muscle, just as all other muscles in upper motor neuron disease, becomes hypertonic and spastic. Bladder capacity is decreased and frequency of urination is uncertain, since even small accumulations of urine may trigger reflex activity that causes the bladder to empty. Incontinence occurs quite often because the brain is not inhibiting bladder function. Residual collections of urine may or may not be a problem, depending on the amount of muscle tone in the bladder.

Lower Motor Neuron Bladder

Disease or injury that affects the spinal cord below the T12 level or affects the motor nerves and reflex arcs supplying the bladder results in a condition called *lower motor neuron bladder* or *atonic bladder*. Multiple sclerosis, Guillain-Barré syndrome, and myelomeningocele can all cause this condition, as can low spinal cord transection or temporary spinal shock after any spinal injury. If only motor nerves or the anterior horns of the spinal cord are affected, only motor activity is nonfunctional. If only sensory fibers or the posterior columns of the spinal cord are damaged, only bladder sensation is absent. If the entire reflex arc is interrupted, both motor supply and sensation will be lost.

In all cases, bladder capacity is increased and the bladder easily becomes overdistended. The sensation of fullness may be lost if sensory fibers are destroyed, and bladder contractions will be weak or absent if motor supply is gone. The patient may experience urinary retention with overflow incontinence and will strain to try to empty the bladder, but will still have residual urine left after voiding.

NURSING INTERVENTIONS IN CARING
FOR A PATIENT WITH NEUROGENIC BLADDER

The nursing approaches that are taken to help the patient with an alteration in urinary elimination depend on the specific pathology that exists. A different approach may be taken for the patient with an UMN bladder, for example, as would be taken for the patient with a LMN bladder. The approach may also vary according to the individual patient's normal pattern of urination, which has been assessed on admission to the health facility, and according to the patient's own wishes. As in all other aspects of nursing, the goals of care and the means used to reach those goals must be acceptable to the patient, or all of the nursing care will be in vain. In many health facilities it is the physician who decides initially on the overall approach to urinary control, and the nurse who carries out that plan, using independent judgment and nursing skills.

Diagnostic Studies

The first decisions about setting goals and an overall plan to regain urinary control are usually based on diagnostic studies performed by the physician or radiologist. Since injuries and disease may cause incomplete or mixed lesions, the type of neurogenic bladder may not be readily apparent. Diagnostic tests help to determine the exact extent of bladder function. An intravenous pyelogram (IVP) may be done to rule out kidney or urethral pathology. Urodynamic studies are performed to measure the bladder capacity and pressure (cystometrogram) and functioning ability of the urethra (urethral pressure profile). Urine is also tested, with specific attention to the presence of large numbers of bacteria and white blood cells, which would indicate the presence of infection. When all of these data have been collected, the physician and nurse can then decide which approaches to achieving urinary control are feasible and most practicable for the patient.

Methods of Controlling Urinary Incontinence

There are several methods of controlling incontinence that are in common use. Some methods that make nursing care easier in a busy hospital unit, such as the indwelling catheter, may not be in the best interest of the patient. Other methods, such as every-2-hour bedpan schedule, which may be very effective for some patients, require a great deal of nursing time and may not be carried out consistently on evening and night shifts or on weekends. A method should be found that can reasonably be carried out with the given staff situation and physical environment and which follows the principles of good nursing practice.

The method that is initially chosen may be used only for a limited period of time and then changed as the patient's condition changes. For example, the stroke patient may have a completely uninhibited bladder with constant incontinence during the acute stage of illness, but may gradually achieve some spontaneous urinary control as the cerebral edema and anoxia begin to subside. The patient with spinal cord transection may initially present with an atonic bladder with dribbling and overdistention during spinal shock and later have a reflex bladder that empties when certain trigger points are touched.

Indwelling catheters. Indwelling catheters are very often inserted in the emergency department of a hospital in order to measure exact hourly urinary output and to prevent overdistention of the bladder. These catheters (usually Foley catheters) are left in place during the acute stage of illness or as long as a patient is unconscious. If when the catheter is removed the patient is found to be incontinent, a decision has to be made about the next course of action. Reinserting the catheter may predispose the patient to certain complications.

The rate of urinary tract infection in patients with indwelling catheters is very high. Gram-negative organisms from the bowel and perineal area are often introduced into the bladder at the time of catheterization. Strict sterile technique and proper disinfection of the meatus can reduce infection via this route. After insertion, pathological organisms can continue to travel up along the catheter into the bladder. Frequent catheter care with a bacteriostatic soap or solution can reduce this type of infection.

The entire drainage system should be airtight, a closed system, or else bacteria can ascend the catheter on air bubbles that rise up to the bladder. You should always take specimens by sterile syringe rather than by disconnecting the tubing. It is important to use a small catheter

(14 or 16F). A small-diameter catheter allows urethral secretions to drain to the outside rather than be trapped in the urethra and serve as a culture medium for bacteria. Large catheters are also more likely to traumatize the urethra on insertion, again predisposing the patient to infection.

Urine should not remain static in the tubing, nor should it be allowed to flow back into the bladder from the tubing. Always keeping the bag and tubing below bladder level and coiling and taping excess tubing on the mattress will prevent these contingencies. Most drainage bags are equipped with one-way valves that prevent urine from flowing back from the collection bag into the tubing. Fluid intake should be increased to 3 or 4 liters, unless contraindicated, to ensure a good flow of urine through the system.

There is some debate over how often an indwelling catheter should be replaced. Latex catheters can only be used for about 1 week, because there is a danger of phosphate deposits forming around the balloon, which break up when the balloon is deflated, resulting in bladder calculi. Silicone catheters are not subject to phosphate deposits and can be left in for long-term use. Silicone catheters have to be replaced only if they become obstructed or if there is a lot of sediment in the tube. The more often a catheter is changed, the greater the chance of infection.

Indwelling catheters are usually taped to the patient's thigh or abdomen. The weight of the bag and tubing constantly pulling on the balloon can cause irritation of the bladder neck. An extra tug on the tubing when a patient is getting in or out of the bed could be enough force to pull the balloon into the urethra or out of the body completely, causing a great deal of damage. Taping the catheter securely with some slack in it will prevent these complications. With a female patient, tape the catheter to the thigh. With a male patient who has a catheter for more than a few days, tape it laterally to the thigh (penis at right angle to the thigh) or up onto the abdomen to prevent pressure on the urethra at the penoscrotal junction, which can result in fistula formation.

When it seems advisable to remove the indwelling catheter, the patient is often placed on a catheter clamping schedule, such as clamping for 4 hours, opening for 10 minutes, and reclamping for 4 hours. While the catheter is open the patient is told to void through the catheter by contracting the abdominal and perineal muscles. This practice is thought to increase pelvic and bladder muscle tone, allowing for better control of urination after the catheter is removed. In fact, however, the effectiveness of the procedure has not been proven, and may even be harmful if the bladder becomes overdistended. Bladder and sphincter tone can usually be regained, except in some lower motor neuron disorders, by removing the catheter and then having the patient do perineal muscle contraction exercises and stop the urinary stream periodically while voiding.

Cystotomy tube. There are some patients who cannot manage without a catheter but who cannot tolerate an indwelling catheter. The presence of the indwelling catheter may cause very painful bladder spasms and urination around the catheter (sometimes seen in multiple sclerosis). In such cases, a suprapubic cystotomy tube is inserted by the physician. Suprapubic bladder drainage is very effective, often more comfortable, and carries less chance of infection. Nursing care involves cleansing around the insertion site, applying sterile dressings, and taping the tube to the abdomen.

Diapering. Diapering incontinent patients, especially females, is a common practice in many nursing homes and even in some hospitals. It is thought that diapering is superior to an indwelling catheter because there is little risk of infection. The practice of diapering, however, brings its own problems. Using standard adult disposable diapers or incontinent pads means leaving the patient lying soaked in urine, often for hours at a time. Not only is this productive of unpleasant odors, but the skin quickly becomes irritated and macerated unless diapers are changed as soon as wet. New adult diaper products are now being produced that are much more absorbent and keep moisture away from the skin; they are more acceptable, but should be used only when other methods have been ruled out. You must consider the psychological effects that diapering may have. For the alert adult, it may be a humiliating, degrading form of treatment that will negatively affect the self-esteem.

Toileting schedules. You may be able to keep patients dry by placing them on the commode or bedpan or giving the urinal at frequent scheduled intervals. This, of course, is not useful for patients who dribble almost constantly, but can be helpful for many patients with some urinary control. The frequency of toileting is determined by the fluid intake and usual frequency of incontinence. You may set the schedule for every 2 to every 4 hours, depending on the patient. Some nurses keep a urinal in place constantly to prevent bed-wetting, but this practice can result in severe irritation of the groin, penis, and inner thighs, and often still results in a wet bed as the urinal moves. Incontinent male patients benefit much more from external catheters.

External catheters. An external or condom-type catheter can be used to control male incontinence. External catheters are made by many companies, and all have slight variations. Basically, they are all

comprised of a flexible plastic condom-like collecting device that is
rolled up over the penis, and some type of elastic tape to secure it (see
Figure 4.1). They can be connected to any standard drainage tubing
and bag. Success with the apparatus depends on correct application.
When the collector is rolled up over the penis, a ½-inch space should be
left between the tip of the penis and the inside of the collector device.

You must take care to prevent the collector from twisting at the
point where it joins the drainage tubing. If the collector becomes twisted,
urine collects around the penis and begins to cause skin breakdown.
This is a very common problem and can only be avoided by careful
positioning of the tubing, usually maintained by taping it laterally to
the thigh.

Circulatory impairment is another hazard. Tape should not be
applied circumferentially since it might constrict the penis, but rather
should be applied in a spiral fashion. Elastic tape must be used to accommodate any swelling, especially if the patient is likely to have
reflexogenic erections. If double-sided elastic tape is being used *inside*
the collector, against the skin, some type of skin protector, such as
Skin Prep (United Surgical), should be used.

Although some hospitals recommend changing the apparatus every
other day, it is safer to change it every day. If there is backflow of urine
over the penis, extensive maceration can occur in 2 days. When you
change the collection device, wash the penis carefully with soap and
water, rinse, and dry thoroughly. Good hygiene will help to prevent
maceration and infection. When used correctly, problems should not
occur, and external collection can go on indefinitely. If the patient is
prone to skin irritation or swelling, this method of controlling incontinence may have to be terminated, or alternated with another
method.

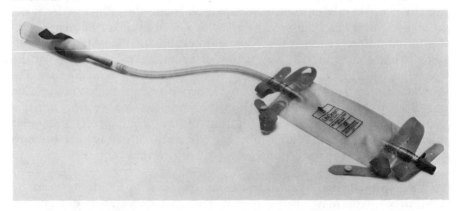

Figure 4.1 Uri-Drain external catheter and leg bag. (Courtesy of Chese-
brough-Ponds, Inc.)

Whichever method you choose to control incontinence, you must then follow up with an appropriate evaluation. Does this method keep the patient dry? Is it likely to cause unnecessary infection? Is the patient satisfied and comfortable with the plan? Is it practical in terms of time and expense? If your evaluation reveals weaknesses in the method, what else could you try that might be better?

An important factor in the success of any nursing intervention for incontinence is continuity of care between shifts of nurses. You can maximize continuity by writing nursing orders which ensure that proper and standardized care will be given. For example, if an indwelling catheter is being used, a few of your orders might be: "Tape catheter up on abdomen, preventing contact between penis and scrotum. Change tape QOD." and "Change catheter every week on Monday, use only size 16F." Other nurses can then follow your orders or adapt them if necessary, and the patient will get better regulated and organized care.

Methods of Promoting Bladder Emptying

Patients with both lower and upper motor neuron bladders may experience difficulty in emptying the bladder of urine. In the LMN bladder, flaccid muscles and weak contractions may result in filling of the bladder to the point of overdistention if nothing is done to intervene. Overdistention of the bladder is an eventuality you must prevent at all costs, since it leads to impaired bladder sensation that could last for months. With any neurogenic bladder, even if some urine is put out, large amounts of residual urine may be left in the bladder. Residual collections can lead not only to overdistention, but also to infection.

Intermittent catheterization. Several measures have been refined that assist the patient in emptying the bladder without resorting to a continuous indwelling catheter. Intermittent catheterization has become a popular and very effective technique in patients who have a good prognosis. Especially useful in spinal cord injuries, this technique is often begun right after the acute stage of illness, when the patient's physical condition has been stabilized. It can be used for the atonic bladder during spinal shock (usually a period of 1 to 3 months) and is continued for a period of time afterward. In this regimen, catheterization is done about every 4 to 6 hours using strict sterile technique. Intake is calculated very carefully to determine the specific frequency with which catheterization needs to be done for an individual patient. The infection rate with intermittent therapy is considerably less than with indwelling catheters, and the patient gains greater freedom without the constant presence of the tube.

In the case of upper motor neuron spinal cord injuries, reflex activity returns to the bladder, and eventually intermittent catheterization will be discontinued and other techniques substituted. Weaning a patient off catheterization involves careful measurement of intake and output, palpation or percussion of bladder size, and measurement of residual urine.

When the patient with an UMN bladder first begins to void by reflex, residual amounts of urine left in the bladder may be quite large. Intermittent catheterization is continued after voidings to measure residual urine and to empty the bladder. The patient palpates or percusses the bladder before catheterization to determine the size of it, and quickly learns to relate the size of the bladder to the amount of urine in it. Gradually, over a period of weeks or months, voiding will be more complete. When residual amounts are less than 50 mℓ, catheterization can be discontinued. The patient should continue to palpate the bladder after voidings to make sure that large residuals do not occur.

The patient with a LMN bladder may be unable to manage without intermittent catheterization. In this case, self-catheterization may be taught, so that bladder complications are minimized, yet the patient can regain a measure of independence. Self-catheterization requires clean rather than sterile technique. The person needs access to soap and water, a catheter, and water soluble lubricant. Washing the hands with soap and water before starting the procedure is recommended. However, if it is not available, commercial antiseptic wipes may be used. Rubber catheters are used and are washed with soap and water between uses. They are stored in a plastic bag or case, and need to be replaced only if they become hard or if they acquire an odor.

The male patient catheterizes himself while sitting or standing. The catheter must be lubricated. The female patient can also do the procedure while sitting or standing, but will initially need a mirror to visualize the meatus. Later the patient can locate the meatus without the aid of a mirror. A woman may not need to lubricate the catheter. With a fluid intake of about 2500 mℓ, the individual may only have to catheterize about every 8 hours.

Stimulation of trigger points. Spontaneous reflex voiding can be accomplished in the patient with a reflex bladder and is one of the methods used after the patient is weaned off intermittent catheterization. Various *trigger points* can be found on the bodies of these individuals, which when touched, stroked, or stretched will stimulate the bladder to contract and voiding to occur. For example, the patient may stroke the inner aspects of the thighs, tap the abdomen, pull on pubic hair, massage the sacrum, or manually stretch the anal sphincter. Different methods will work for different individuals and can only be discovered by trial and error. Once patients have found how to trigger urination, they need only learn how often to do it, by assessing fluid intake, palpating bladder size, and being alert to symptoms of a distended bladder, such as perspiration, restlessness, a chilly feeling, or vague anxiety.

Credé maneuver. The Credé method of emptying the bladder consists of manual expression of urine by applying pressure over the suprapubic area (see Figure 4.2). It is useful in lower motor neuron disease with a bladder that has no reflex emptying. The patient or nurse places a hand over the suprapubic area and exerts downward pressure. It is most effective if the patient is sitting up and leaning forward, allowing the anatomical structures and gravity to assist. This maneuver is very safe and easily performed.

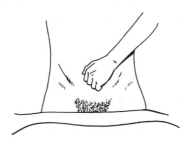

Figure 4.2 The Credé method of emptying the bladder.

Medications. Several classifications of drugs have been used in treatment of neurogenic bladder. Cholinergic (parasympathomimetic) drugs such as bethanechol chloride (Urecholine) elicit or strengthen bladder contractions and have therefore been useful in aiding bladder emptying in a variety of conditions. Anticholinergic (parasympathetic blocker) medications such as propantheline bromide (Pro-Banthine) reduce the tonicity of the bladder and are often given for bladder spasms and urinary frequency (especially seen in multiple sclerosis). Imipramine (Tofranil) has been used successfully in spastic bladders because of its relaxation effect on bladder muscle. Ephedrine, an adrenergic drug, works specifically to stimulate the sphincters, thus reducing incontinence. Since all these drugs have autonomic effects, they work on other parts of the body as well as the bladder, and therefore warrant careful reading of the drug literature and assessment for possible side effects. Pharmacologic agents are never used independently to treat neurogenic bladder, but are one part of the overall plan for management of urinary control.

Complications

Many of the nursing and medical interventions attempted in patients with neurogenic bladder will be dogged by complications; in some cases, none of these approaches will be successful. Many patients with neurogenic bladder will at some time during their disability suffer from urinary infection. While this may be inhibited by forcing fluids and keeping the urine acid by drinking cranberry juice, it is also true that in some cases infection will occur and may ascend to the kidneys, causing serious problems and perhaps even leading to death. Some patients will also be plagued with urinary calculi, in spite of increased fluid intake. The possibility also exists that hypertrophy of the walls of a reflex bladder may lead to vesicoureteral reflux and hydronephrosis. Those for whom none of the nursing or medical interventions work may have to have surgery, such as widening of the bladder neck, urethrotomy, or even urinary diversion (ileal conduit or continent vesicotomy).

It is important for the nurse to be familiar with the alternatives available to the patient with neurogenic bladder and to have a basic knowledge of when various interventions can be expected to work and how they work.

BOWEL PATHOLOGY

Normal defecation usually occurs as pressure is exerted against the rectal walls, causing a reflex contraction of the rectum and relaxation of the anal sphincter. When disease or injury affects the sacral segments of the spinal cord and surrounding nerves (lower motor neuron disease), reflex action is lost and the external sphincter relaxes; the patient loses control over excretion and may have continual incontinence.

If the damage occurs higher in the cord, the reflex arcs remain intact but uninhibited (similar to the reflex bladder) and the patient experiences periodic reflex emptying of the bowel. Injury or disease that affects only the posterior roots or columns (sensory tracts) destroys the pressure sensation in the rectum that normally stimulates emptying action, resulting in retention of stool.

NURSING INTERVENTIONS FOR ABNORMAL
BOWEL EMPTYING

Monitoring bowel elimination and promoting normal defecation is a nursing responsibility that takes a great deal of nursing time. Although bowel training programs may initially require a large investment of time, the long-term results will be a savings of nursing time once incontinence or constipation has been brought under control. A successful bowel program also enables the disabled patient to progress to other aspects of rehabilitation.

Methods of Controlling Bowel Incontinence

Fecal incontinence bags.   Some hospitals and nursing homes have experimented with commercially produced fecal collection bags. These bags resemble ostomy bags, with an adhesive face plate that is supposed to adhere to the skin around the anus. Unfortunately, they have been rather unsuccessful. It is difficult to get a good skin seal in the perineal area, so the bags are frequently found lying in the bed. If the bag *is* well attached, it must be pulled off the skin and replaced when soiled, thereby irritating the skin and contributing to breakdown.

Bowel cleansing routine.   Rather than having feces passing or oozing periodically from the rectum, it is often better, especially for the unconscious patient, to give a cleansing enema every other day to evacuate the lower colon completely at one time. The patient may then stay clean until the next enema. This regimen is much like that followed by the colostomate, who irrigates the colostomy every morning and then does not need to wear a bag. You should determine the frequency of enemas by the patient's premorbid bowel habits, if known, and by the frequency of incontinence. It may be possible to accomplish the same result by using suppositories rather than enemas. A Dulcolax suppository may stimulate bowel emptying and may be enough of a stimulus to empty the bowel completely.

Methods of Promoting Bowel Emptying

Retention of stool in the lower colon is seen in patients with long-term debilitating diseases such as multiple sclerosis and Parkinson's disease, as well as in patients with cerebrovascular accidents or spinal cord injuries. Stool that is retained in the lower colon continues to undergo dehydration and becomes hard and difficult to expel. Several simple nursing interventions can help to prevent constipation and establish routine bowel habits.

Diet. Encouraging a patient to eat a diet high in residue and fiber will be of enormous help. Foods such as bran or whole-wheat grain cereals and breads and fresh fruit will provide bulk to the stool and stimulate defecation. Fluids provide moisture and lubrication for the feces and should be increased to 3000 or 4000 mℓ if there are no contraindications such as cardiac decompensation. Prune juice is a natural laxative which also helps keep the stools soft.

Too often nurses leave all diet planning to the dietitian and only concern themselves with it when a problem arises. If you wait until a patient is very constipated to think of giving prune juice or increasing bulk in the diet, you have waited too long. After assessing the patient's elimination needs and normal pattern, you should immediately begin to plan how to prevent problems in constipation-prone patients. Include nursing orders in your plan, such as "Make sure a high-fiber cereal or bread is included on breakfast menu, and a fruit salad for dinner everyday." Or, "Give 150 mℓ prune juice with breakfast OD." Preventing constipation is much easier than treating it.

Activity and exercise. Walking is one of the best forms of exercise but is often difficult or impossible for the neurologically impaired. Those who can walk should certainly be encouraged to do so, since this exercise also helps to propel the stool and strengthens abdominal and pelvic muscles needed in the act of defecation. If locomotion is not possible, stationary exercises can be employed. Younger patients can perhaps do sit-ups for muscle strengthening. Older patients may only be able to do isometric muscle tightening of the abdominal and gluteal muscles. Completely paralyzed patients will even derive benefit from being turned and receiving passive exercises.

Medications. Stool softeners or wetting agents are valuable in preventing constipation and straining. If too much straining occurs, hemorrhoids may result, adding to the patient's plight. Stool softeners permit water and fatty substances to pass into the stools, thus making them soft but formed. These are very safe drugs and can be used indefinitely.

Cathartics or laxatives are effective in emptying the bowel, but should not be relied upon for long-term use. They can cause chronic irritation of the bowel leading to diarrhea, or since they lead to loss of muscle tone, can actually complicate the constipation problem.

Enemas and digital removal of fecal impactions. Enemas, like cathartics, should not be depended on for long periods of time, unless absolutely necessary. Enemas have many of the same drawbacks as cathartics and are time consuming. If a patient develops a fecal impaction, however, enemas will be necessary to alleviate the problem. Fecal impaction results from prolonged retention of stool until a mass accumulates that is too large to pass through the anus. This mass is very hard and dry and irritates the colonic lining, often stimulating the production of liquid and mucus that is passed around the impaction together with some liquid stool.

If oil retention or cleansing enemas do not soften and break up the impaction, it may be necessary for you to manually break it up and remove it by inserting a gloved finger gently into the rectum. Rectal stimulation of any type should be avoided in a patient suspected of having increased intracranial pressure, since this action can further increase the pressure. If not contraindicated, a patient who has not had a bowel movement in 3 days should always be checked for the possibility of fecal impaction.

Bowel retraining. A program of bowel retraining should be instituted for any patient who has a good physical prognosis. It can be especially successful in patients with reflex bowel activity but can also be instituted for those individuals with lower motor neuron disease. The previous measures of adequate diet and exercise are included. In addition, encourage the patient to set a specific time of the day for bowel elimination, usually after breakfast, or at least after a warm cup of tea or coffee in the morning. The meal or warm fluid helps to stimulate peristalsis. The patient should then insert a Dulcolax or glycerin suppository, wait 30 minutes if possible, then sit on the toilet and try to expel feces without straining. Leaning forward or sitting with the feet on a low footstool will help to increase intraabdominal pressure.

After a few weeks, it may be possible for the person with reflex activity to discontinue the suppository and thereafter stimulate reflex emptying by massaging the anal sphincter with a gloved finger inserted 1 to 1½ inches and rotated a few times. The individual with no reflex arc activity will derive no benefit from sphincter stimulation and may continue to require suppositories, and can also apply external pressure to the abdomen in an attempt to empty the bowel completely and prevent intermittent soiling.

As with interventions for urinary problems, the approaches to bowel disturbances described above may not work perfectly for all patients. Not every patient fits the textbook picture or responds in the expected way, but with some variations and creative combinations of therapy, a satisfactory routine can be worked out.

AUTONOMIC HYPERREFLEXIA

Autonomic hyperreflexia (or dysreflexia) is a very serious syndrome that may develop in a patient with a spinal cord injury above the T4 level (the sympathetic nerve outflow) after spinal shock wears off. Excessive sensory stimulation, usually from a full bowel or bladder or from stimulation of skin in the perineal area (decubiti, excessive pressure, etc.), sets off an uninhibited sympathetic response with release of norepinephrine. The response is uninhibited because the spinal cord can no longer pass along messages to evoke compensatory mechanisms below the level of the lesion. The norepinephrine causes general body vasoconstriction and can dangerously increase the blood pressure. Eventually, pressure receptors in the carotid sinus and aortic arch interpret the hypertension and send out messages causing bradycardia and vasodilation above the cord lesion.

The typical picture of a hyperreflexia episode begins with a headache, then paroxysmal hypertension and fast pulse, followed by diaphoresis and flushing of the skin above the lesion, and bradycardia. Any patient with a high spinal cord lesion should be observed carefully if headache begins. If allowed to progress unchecked, this type of crisis can result in increased intracranial pressure, cerebral hemorrhage, or myocardial infarction.

Management of the syndrome consists of removing the cause. Check for obstruction of a catheter that might have led to a distended bladder, for the presence of a fecal impaction, or for anything causing pressure on the perineal area. If the cause is removed, the condition will subside quickly and require no treatment. Setting the patient up in high Fowler's position will help to reduce intracranial pressure. Blood pressure should be checked every 5 minutes; if the pressure does not start to come down, intravenous antihypertensives may be given. In a patient prone to develop hyperreflexia, removal of impactions or enemas for any reason should be done only after an anesthetic ointment is applied to the anus to 1 inch inside the rectum.

NURSING CONCERN FOR ELIMINATION PROBLEMS

Elimination difficulties have a great impact on the patient and warrant the use of scientific thought and the concerted efforts of the health team to find satisfactory solutions. Elimination is one of our most personal and private concerns, generally not discussed with others. Patients have their most intimate bodily functions brought out into conversation and even into the nurses' view. There is often little concern for privacy and modesty. Patients are often embarrassed by elimination problems and may despair of ever controlling them or living normally again. They may feel as if they have regressed to childhood or as if they are dirty. So it is worth giving our time and attention to solving or improving urination and defecation difficulties. We need to assess, plan, intervene, and then evaluate, just as we do for problems of oxygenation or communication, to improve the quality of life for our patients.

**EXAMPLES OF NURSING DIAGNOSES
RELATED TO ELIMINATION**

Inability to empty bladder completely related to loss of muscle tone; urine residuals above 100 mℓ.

Urinary incontinence related to uninhibited sphincter action.

Anxiety related to continuing urinary incontinence.

Altered self-concept related to wearing a urinary appliance.

Potential for urinary complications due to low fluid intake.

Lack of knowledge related to perineal hygiene.

Alteration in bowel elimination related to change in diet; has small, hard stool every 3 days.

Alteration in bowel elimination related to spinal cord injury; has small unpredictable spontaneous bowel movements.

Bowel incontinence related to cerebral damage.

REFERENCES

Alpers, Bernard, and Elliott L. Mancall, *Clinical Neurology*. Philadelphia: F. A. Davis Company, 1971.

Barber, Janet Miller, and others, *Adult and Child Care*. St. Louis: The C. V. Mosby Company, 1977.

Beber, Charles R., "Freedom for the Incontinent," *American Journal of Nursing*, 80, no. 3 (March 1980), p. 482.

Boyarsky, Saul, and others, *Care of the Patient with Neurogenic Bladder*. Boston: Little, Brown and Company, 1979.

Brunner, Lillian Sholtis, and Doris Smith Suddarth, *Textbook of Medical-Surgical Nursing*. Philadelphia: J. B. Lippincott Company, 1980.

Catanzaro, Marci, "Nursing Care of the Person with MS," *American Journal of Nursing*, 80, no. 2 (February 1980), p. 286.

Felder, Lauren, "Neurogenic Bladder Dysfunction," *Journal of Neurosurgical Nursing*, 11, no. 2 (June 1979), p. 94.

Feustel, Delycia, "Autonomic Hyperreflexia," *American Journal of Nursing*, 76, no. 2 (February 1976), p. 228.

Jameson, Robert Morpeth, *Management of the Urological Patient*. New York: Churchill Livingstone, 1976.

Kinney, Anna Belle, and others, "Urethral Catheterization," *Geriatric Nursing*, 1, no. 4 (November–December 1980), p. 258.

Whyte, John F., and Nancy A. Thistle, "Male Incontinence: The Inside Story on External Collection," *Nursing 76*, 6, no. 9 (September 1976), p. 66.

Zankel, Harry T., *Stroke Rehabilitation*, Springfield, Ill.: Charles C Thomas, Publisher, 1971.

5

Alterations in Respiratory Function

Respiratory impairment is not uncommon among people with neurologic problems. Since the nervous system stimulates respirations and keeps the muscles of respiration working, it is not surprising that difficulty breathing and inadequate ventilation are results of neurologic disease and can be causes of death in the victims of nervous system disorders. Nursing care that relieves respiratory difficulty and prevents pulmonary complications can improve the quality of life for many patients.

NORMAL RESPIRATORY MECHANISMS

The cerebrum, brainstem, nerve pathways and the muscles they innervate, and certain chemoreceptor cells are all involved in neurologic control of respiration. The cerebral cortex functions in the voluntary aspects of breathing, giving us conscious control of our respirations. The medulla and pons in the brainstem are the primary neural areas for control of involuntary respiration. In fact, the medulla is usually referred to as the *respiratory center*. It contains neurons which regulate both inspiration and expiration; it receives incoming messages from the spinal cord, pons, cortex, and from the various chemoreceptors, all reporting on the need for changes in inspiration and expiration; it sends out messages to the muscles of respiration, telling them to contract or relax.

The pons receives messages from the lungs themselves as they inflate and deflate. The pons passes on the information to the medulla and the medulla passes back instructions for the lungs. This cycle is known as the Hering-Breuer reflex. When the lungs inflate, the reflex is stimulated, and the brainstem tells the lungs when to stop inflating and begin deflating. The reflex is again triggered upon deflation, and the brainstem tells the lungs when to stop deflating and again start inflating.

There are chemoreceptors in the medulla which monitor the pH of the cerebrospinal fluid (CSF). The changes that are detected in the pH result in changes in the respiratory rate or depth. For example, if the chemoreceptors pick up a falling pH in the CSF, the respiratory center will be stimulated and respirations will increase. Chemoreceptors located in the carotid arteries and the aortic arch respond to changes in arterial oxygen, carbon dioxide, or pH and send messages to the medulla via the glossopharyngeal and vagus nerves, respectively, stimulating a change in respirations.

The muscles of respiration are a necessary part of the ventilation process. By contracting and then relaxing, they serve to bring air into the chest and let it out again, and they enable a person to cough effectively. The diaphragm is a powerful muscle that contracts when stimulated by the phrenic nerve and moves downward, increasing the size of the chest cavity. The intercostal muscles pull the ribs up and outward when they contract. When respiratory demands are increased, accessory muscles of the neck or abdomen may be used to help in the act of breathing.

As the chest size increases on inspiration, intraalveolar pressure becomes slightly negative (less than atmospheric pressure), and air is pulled into the alveoli from the bronchial tree. The pressure then equalizes and expiration begins. The alveoli have a constant tendency to collapse, because of their natural elasticity and because of the high surface tension of the fluid that lines them. The alveoli therefore secrete a substance known as *pulmonary surfactant*, a lipoprotein substance that markedly reduces the surface tension of the respiratory fluids and keeps the alveoli open under normal conditions.

NEUROLOGIC DISORDERS THAT INVOLVE RESPIRATORY IMPAIRMENT

Respiratory function can be affected in several different ways in the presence of neurologic disease. Cerebral damage may interfere with voluntary control of respiration. Brainstem trauma can eliminate or hamper involuntary respiratory controls and can be rapidly fatal. Neuromuscular disorders can weaken the respiratory muscles or the cough response, thus interfering with the mechanical aspects of breathing. The gag reflex may be paralyzed, leading to aspiration. Specific disorders will be discussed in relation to their effect on respiration.

Coma

Regardless of the cause of the coma, respiratory care is essential. Comatose patients frequently die from respiratory complications due to aspiration of food, retained secretions which obstruct the airways, or from respiratory infections. Food aspiration often occurs when tube feedings are given improperly. Secretions are retained in any patient who does not cough effectively. The secretions become very thick and obstruct the airways, leading to atelectasis and pneumonia. Infection can also result from long-term mechanical ventilation or from tracheostomies performed to open the airway. Bacteria may be harbored in respiratory equipment and will frequently cause disease in debilitated and critically ill patients.

Myasthenia Gravis

Myasthenia gravis is a disease in which it is believed that antibodies are produced against a person's own neuromuscular junctions. Acetylcholine is normally released from a motor nerve ending, then crosses the synapse to trigger a contraction in the muscle. In myasthenia gravis, this transmission does not take place normally. Any voluntary muscle may be affected, the most common being the muscles used for chewing, swallowing, moving the eyes, and breathing. Muscle weakness may be slight or severe and gets progressively worse as the muscle is being used.

Symptoms may become much more severe during times of stress or infection, precipitating a crisis situation. During periods of crisis the patient's vital capacity may steadily decrease as muscular weakness increases, atelectasis and hypoxia ensue, and finally a tracheostomy and mechanical ventilation will be needed. The situation may be compounded by the fact that the anticholinesterase drugs used in treatment of myasthenia cause excessive secretions that the patient cannot handle.

Guillain-Barré Syndrome

Acute infectious polyneuritis, or Guillain-Barré syndrome, involves viral inflammation of the spinal and cranial nerve roots with accompanying weakness or flaccid paralysis of individual muscle groups. The paralysis is classically ascending in nature, but may often affect the upper extremities and trunk or head first. Difficulty swallowing followed by aspiration leads to pulmonary problems. Weakness of the respiratory muscles brings about a reduction in the vital capacity which can lead to respiratory failure and death if not treated.

Poliomyelitis

There are two forms of polio that interfere with respiratory function. Bulbar poliomyelitis is characterized by viral inflammation of the ninth to twelfth cranial nerves which affects swallowing and paralyzes the larynx. Involvement of the medulla may eliminate the normal respiratory stimuli. Spinal poliomyelitis, with paralysis only of the spinal nerves, weakens the respiratory muscles and prohibits coughing. Both forms of polio may need to be treated with mechanical ventilation. Patients who recover from this disease may be left with residual respiratory problems such as reduced vital capacity, together with decreased respiratory reserves and monotonous, even respirations that predispose to atelectasis and infection.

Cervical Spinal Cord Injuries

Lesions in the spinal cord above the C4 level are often fatal, but some patients may survive if maintained on a respirator. Since all of the respiratory muscles are paralyzed, these patients will probably always be dependent on mechanical ventilation for as long as they live.

Lesions that are sustained below C4 have a better prognosis from a respiratory standpoint because the phrenic nerve is still intact and can stimulate movement of the diaphragm. Depending on the level of the lesion, all or just some of the intercostal muscles may be paralyzed, thus limiting movement of the rib cage. However, accessory muscles in the neck and shoulders can compensate for the paralyzed intercostals. One of the most serious problems for the quadriplegic is the inability to cough effectively due to paralysis of the abdominal and respiratory muscles. Also, in the acute period after the trauma, paralytic ileus and gastric distention may prevent the diaphragm from descending normally and therefore contribute to the problem of hypoventilation.

Head Injury

Head injuries can alter respiration by several means. Direct trauma to the cerebrum or brainstem can interrupt respiratory control. Such trauma often leads to increased intracranial pressure, which may interfere with blood supply to the respiratory centers. Head injuries with concomitant facial injuries may cause an obstructed airway, or the airway may be blocked by secretions. Cerebral trauma that alters the level of consciousness usually results in alveolar hypoventilation due to shallow respirations. All these possibilities can ultimately progress to respiratory failure or respiratory arrest, and together they account for a high mortality rate among head-injured patients.

Increased intracranial pressure. Hypoxia develops in head injury cases for any one of the reasons mentioned above. As hypoxia progresses, cell membranes become increasingly permeable, and intracellular and intravascular fluid move into interstitial spaces, creating cerebral edema. At the same time, hypercapnia is also developing, with high carbon dioxide levels acting to dilate cerebral blood vessels and increase blood flow. This combination of effects from lack of oxygen and too much carbon dioxide can therefore lead to elevated intracranial pressure from cerebral edema.

Increasing volume within the cranium inevitably puts so great a pressure on brain tissue that blood supply to vital areas is impaired. If the respiratory centers are not receiving adequate blood, they are also not getting adequate oxygen, and these delicate tissues begin to break down and eventually stop functioning.

Acute pulmonary edema. This problem frequently follows increased intracranial pressure. When intracranial pressure rises, the sympathetic nervous system stimulates general body vasoconstriction with increased blood vessel resistance and hypertension. Cardiac output increases as a result of hypertension, and more blood is pushed to the lungs. Increasing permeability of pulmonary blood vessels due to anaerobic metabolism in the lung cells contributes to the process by allowing fluid to move into the alveoli. Thus, a process that began because of hypoxia ends in even greater hypoxia because of fluid pooling in the lungs.

Shock lung syndrome. Lack of oxygen to the central nervous system appears to be one of the many causes of *adult respiratory distress syndrome* (ARDS), more commonly known as *shock lung syndrome*. Comprising this syndrome are pulmonary capillary vasoconstriction, increased capillary permeability with fluid leakage into the alveoli, physiologic shunting of unoxygenated blood, and finally acidosis. Surfactant is either not produced in adequate amounts or is inactivated, causing loss of compliance and atelectasis. Eventually, hyaline membranes form in the alveoli, interfering with gas absorption. Pneumonia is usually the end stage before death from hypoxemia or heart failure. Shock lung carries a high mortality rate, but can often be prevented by care that increases pulmonary and cerebral oxygenation.

MAINTAINING LUNG VENTILATION

Indications for Mechanical Ventilation of Neurologic Patients

The decision to institute mechanical ventilation is a medical one, but the observations and judgment of the nurse contribute valuable input to the decision-making process. You may be the first person to recognize increasing breathlessness, cyanosis, or a change in vital signs. When doing routine assessments you may identify a change in the respiratory pattern, or a change in level of consciousness. Complaints of a headache or pupillary changes may alert you to increasing intracranial pressure. Early recognition of danger signs and appropriate reporting on your part may mean fast help for a patient with impending respiratory difficulties.

Respirators are used as part of the treatment of increased intracranial pressure. The patient who is put on a respirator can be mechanically *hyperventilated* to bring about respiratory alkalosis. This is desirable with cerebral edema and increased pressure because it reduces cerebral circulation and thus decreases intracranial pressure. Hyperventilation is used in conjunction with osmotic diuretics and corticosteroids in treating elevated pressure medically.

Your observations of ataxic or Cheyne-Stokes respirations may contribute to the physician's decision to use a respirator. Patients whose respirations are very irregular or undependable may need mechanical ventilation to keep their blood gases at safe levels. Paralysis of respiratory muscles, seen in many neuromuscular conditions or spinal cord injury, may necessitate using a respirator until muscular function returns, vital capacity is adequate, and blood gases are stable.

Shock lung syndrome can be prevented in many susceptible patients and can be treated with mechanical ventilation set at *positive end expiratory pressure* (PEEP). PEEP prevents alveoli from collapsing or filling with fluid by maintaining positive pressure even during expiration.

Types of Respirators

There are many varieties of respirators, the broadest classification being negative or positive pressure types. Negative pressure respirators are the tank types that enclose the patient's body and pull air into the lungs as the chest wall is pulled outward. They replace the patient's own muscular effort and are useful in neuromuscular disorders. The most familiar negative pressure respirator is the iron lung, famous for its use during polio epidemics. These machines are seldom used today because they immobilize the patient and make nursing care difficult.

Positive pressure respirators push air into the lungs under pressure. Although the excess pressure may cause problems, this type of respirator is more practical from a nursing care standpoint. Positive pressure respirators also come in three varieties: volume cycled, pressure cycled, or time cycled.

Volume-cycled respirators deliver a preset tidal volume to the patient's lungs. The pressure used to deliver each inspiration may vary, but the patient will always get the same tidal volume or else an alarm will go off. For patients on long-term respirator therapy, this type of machine is best because you know exactly how much air the patient is getting, and lung compliance can be maintained. These machines are also more versatile, offering more options and settings to individualize care.

Pressure-cycled respirators are commonly used for short-term or intermittent therapy or for portable use (see Figure 5.1). They push air into the lungs until a preset pressure is reached, but there is no guarantee that your patient is receiving a desirable tidal volume. If the patient fights the machine or is very restless, the pressure level can be reached before an adequate volume has been delivered. If the lungs are becoming less and less compliant over time, you may not be aware of it because the respirator will still terminate inspiration at the set pressure, regardless of volume.

Time-cycled respirators are most frequently used for infants. They

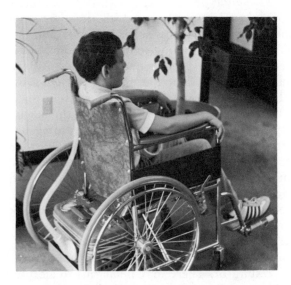

Figure 5.1 A portable G. S. Bantam respirator allows a patient who is respirator dependent to be up and around (Courtesy of Thompson Respiration Products, Inc., 1680 Range, Boulder, Colorado.)

deliver air for a preset time period, determining tidal volume by the length of inspiratory time and the flow rate of the air.

Nursing Responsibilities in Caring for a Patient on a Respirator

Nursing a patient on a respirator can be a frightening experience at first, but a good grasp of certain basic responsibilities can make the experience less overwhelming. First, you must be aware of certain settings and features of the respirator with which you are working. Find out if the patient is on assisted, controlled, or intermittent mandatory ventilation.

Assisted ventilation permits the patient to initiate respirations, but once the patient begins to inhale, the respirator is triggered to deliver the preset volume or pressure. With this system, the patient determines the respiratory rate, but the machine determines the respiratory depth and length of each inspiration.

Controlled ventilation exists when the respirator independently initiates respirations and respiratory volume, thus controlling both rate and depth of breathing. The patient has no control over respirations at all. A combination of assisted and controlled ventilation may also be used to assure a minimum number of respirations if the patient's own rate falls below a preset level.

Intermittent mandatory ventilation (IMV) is a more recent type of respiratory control which can be used all the time or just to wean a patient off the respirator. On this setting, the patient is forced to take a certain number of breaths at a given tidal volume, but in between the machine-forced breaths the patient may spontaneously initiate respirations and may determine their depth. The patient's own respiratory muscles are always doing some work in this system of control, making it easier later for the patient to be weaned from the machine.

The settings for respiratory rate, tidal volume or pressure, and oxygen concentration should be checked periodically to make sure they have not been moved. The physician and respiratory therapist decide on the settings and change them as the patient's condition warrants. Other settings for sighing, expiratory pressure, sensitivity, and so on, are also set by the respiratory therapists and are monitored closely by them. Respiratory therapists have taken over the job of monitoring the respirators, leaving nurses to monitor the patient.

You should know the significance of various alarms that are safety factors on the respirator. There may be alarms to alert you when a preset volume or pressure is not being reached, or to warn you that pressure has increased or has dropped below normal. The alarms only tell you basically what is wrong; you have to find out what is causing the problem. Your observations will usually help you to discover if the problem lies with the patient (for example, fighting the forced rate, obstruction by a mucus plug) or in the machine (disconnected tubing, etc.).

Observations and nursing assessment are essential in determining if the respirator-dependent patient is being adequately ventilated. Every hour or every few hours you will have to auscultate breath sounds in both lungs, listening for evidence of uniform aeration, and for abnormal sounds. If the patient has an endotracheal tube it could slip into the right mainstem bronchus, which is more in line with the trachea, leaving the left lung unventilated. This can be easily diagnosed by auscultation.

Look carefully and frequently at the patient's color. Cyanosis can alert you to hypoventilation. Restlessness and agitation may point to poor oxygenation or inappropriate respirator settings. Evaluation of arterial blood gases by the nurse, respiratory therapist, and physician can help to point out the need for ventilatory changes.

Keep an eye on the tubing between the patient and the respirator. The warm, moist air that is used to keep the patient's secretions moist condenses quickly in this tubing and collects in the dependent portions of the tube. The water collection interferes with gas delivery and may inadvertently be tipped into the patient's airway. Empty the tubing whenever you see water collecting.

Finally, make sure that a hand ventilator such as an Ambu-bag is kept at the bedside to be used in case of machine dysfunction or electrical failure. If you are in doubt about whether the machine is functioning properly, you will always be able to ventilate the patient manually.

Nursing Management of Patient Problems Due to Mechanical Ventilation

Although a respirator solves some of the patient's problems, it can also create new ones. One of the first difficulties that may be encountered is if the patient fights against the respirator. Fighting or bucking can occur if a patient is able to breathe at all spontaneously and attempts to overcome the respirations that are forced by the machine. This may set off the high-pressure alarm. Someone who is able to hear and understand you may relax if you encourage breathing-in every time the machine inspiratory cycle starts. If the fighting continues, the patient's lungs will not be inflated adequately, and the physician may have to sedate or paralyze the patient with Pavulon.

A decrease in cardiac output can be a serious problem for neurologic patients. Positive pressure exerted by the respirator, especially if set on PEEP, decreases venous return to the heart, thus lowering stroke volume and cardiac output. Blood pressure falls, urine output may decrease, and level of consciousness may suffer if the body does not compensate for the problem by increasing tone in the peripheral veins. People with neurologic disorders are often unable to compensate and require medical treatment such as vasopressors and volume expanders to bring up the cardiac output. You must monitor the blood pressure carefully in order to detect problems early in the process.

Putting a patient on a ventilator is supposed to prevent hypoventilation and atelectasis, but both problems can sometimes occur because of the ventilator or in spite of it. Any patient with thick secretions can develop mucous plugs that obstruct the bronchioles and cause alveoli to collapse. Monotonous, even respirations also predispose the patient to atelectasis. If the person is on a respirator with a sigh device, it can be set to make the patient sigh several times an hour just as normal lungs do. These deep breaths can prevent atelectasis. If there is no sigh mechanism, you can hyperinflate the lungs with a hand ventilator (Ambu-bag). Turning and positioning the patient frequently prevents secretions from becoming stagnant and relieves pressure on lung tissue.

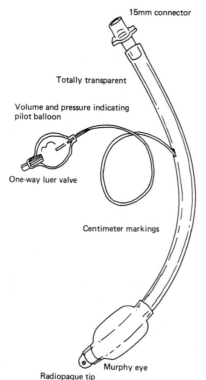

15mm connector

Totally transparent

Volume and pressure indicating
pilot balloon

One-way luer valve

Centimeter markings

Murphy eye

Radiopaque tip

Figure 5.2 Endotracheal tubes. (Courtesy of Shiley Sales Corporation, Irvine, Ca.)

MAINTAINING A PATENT AIRWAY

Patients who have copious secretions blocking their airways or who have paralysis of the pharynx or larynx or facial injuries accompanying head injury require special care to maintain the patency of their airways. In some cases, the lungs may be functioning normally, and it is only the upper airway that needs attention, as in the instance of stroke patients who cannot handle their secretions. In other situations, the upper airway may be normal, but if the lungs are not functioning adequately and need artificial ventilation, an artificial airway may be needed to give access to mechanical ventilation.

Oropharyngeal Airways

The small plastic artificial airways that can be found in any good emergency kit are oropharyngeal airways, designed to lie over the tongue and permit passage of air into the pharynx. They keep the tongue from obstructing the throat, they have a passage that allows the patient to breathe through the device, and they make it easier to suction the mouth and throat. In emergency situations, a plastic airway can be used to keep the airway patent until a better system can be instituted.

Endotracheal Tubes

Endotracheal tubes (see Figure 5.2) can be inserted through either the nose or mouth and they extend down into the trachea. The length of the tube allows it to bypass a paralyzed pharynx or larynx and places it close to the bronchi to make deep suctioning easier. If the tube is inserted through the mouth a bite block must also be used to prevent the patient from biting the soft plastic. Ventilator tubing can be attached to the endotracheal tube if mechanical ventilation is needed. An inflatable cuff can be put around the distal end of the tube to close off the trachea for the purpose of preventing aspiration. When the cuff is inflated, it also provides a barrier between the lungs and the external environment so that when a respirator is being used, air does not escape up the trachea. This type of airway should not be used for more than a few days because it can cause pressure necrosis.

Tracheostomy

For long-term airway maintenance or mechanical ventilation, a tracheostomy is the mode of choice. It bypasses any obstructions in the upper airway, provides easy access to bronchial secretions, and can be used for an indefinite length of time. It may be used only as an airway, or may be an access route for mechanical ventilation.

Tracheostomy care.   Tracheostomy tubes are made of silver, nylon, or plastic. They may be cuffed (see Figure 5.3) or uncuffed, depending on the patient's needs. There are two parts to most tubes, an outer cannula and an inner cannula. The outer cannula should be changed every few days to once a week; the inner cannula is removed for cleaning about every 4 hours. Some plastic tubes do not have inner cannulas and may therefore need to be changed more frequently.

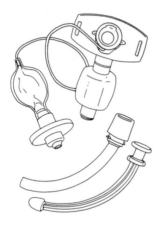

Figure 5.3 Low-pressure cuffed tracheostomy tube with pressure relief valve. (Courtesy of Shiley Sales Corporation, Irvine, Ca.)

Suctioning.   Suctioning of a tracheostomy should be done at least every 4 hours (when the inner cannula is being cleaned) but may be necessary much more frequently. Whenever you hear noisy, moist respirations or the patient becomes dyspneic or cyanotic, suctioning is indicated. You must also suction before deflating the cuff if there is one. Because suctioning removes oxygen from the airways, it must be done only for short periods of time, 10 to 15 seconds at the most, with a 3-minute interval before suctioning again. Waiting to actually begin suctioning until the catheter is as far down as you want it prevents unnecessary removal of oxygen.

Patients who are on respirators should be given extra oxygen and lung inflation prior to and following suctioning. Turn the oxygen concentration up to 100% for 1 minute before and after suctioning, and push the button to sigh the patient a few times (or hyperinflate the patient with a manual bag ventilator). Hyperinflation counteracts any alveolar collapse brought on by suctioning.

Humidification.   A patient with a tracheostomy no longer has the upper airways to warm and humidify inspired air. Giving oxygen through the tracheostomy without giving humidity would soon result in irritated mucous membranes and dried thick secretions. Humidity must be supplied artificially, through such devices as a tracheostomy collar (see Figure 5.4) or through a humidifier attached to the respirator. If secretions are very tenacious, extra moisture can be added by instilling 2 to 5 mℓ of normal saline into the tracheostomy right before suctioning. The saline loosens secretions and induces vigorous coughing.

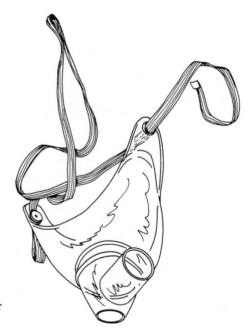

Figure 5.4 Tracheostomy collar or mask.

Communication.   If your patient is alert and able to communicate, you will have to devise a method of communication that fits the situation. A patient with a tracheostomy cannot talk because air now enters the respiratory tree below the level of the vocal cords. If your patient is not on a respirator and is able to tolerate closing the tracheostomy for a few seconds, a finger can be placed over the opening while a few words are spoken. However, most patients are unable to talk at all and will have to communicate with gestures, lipreading, or writing on a Magic Slate.

Problems due to tracheostomy. Two problems associated with tracheostomy are erosion of the trachea and infection. Infection can occur at the incision site, just as with any wound. The infection rate is high because the wound is constantly being irritated by the tracheostomy tube, because secretions collect around the tube, and because these patients are usually very ill and have low resistance. The incidence and severity of infection may be minimized by keeping the wound area free of secretions. It is usually better to dispense with any dressing around the tracheostomy tube after initial bleeding has stopped. Dressings may hide secretions and serve as a culture medium.

Bacteria may enter through the tracheostomy and infect the lower bronchial tree. Patients on mechanical ventilation are especially infection prone because the respirator tubings, which are moist and warm, may incubate bacteria and then deliver them to the lungs. Every time a patient is suctioned there is a chance of contamination of the bronchial tree through a break in technique. Pulmonary infections can be prevented to some degree by making sure that the respirator tubing is changed frequently (every 24 to 48 hours) by the respiratory therapists and by using meticulous suctioning technique.

Tracheal erosion is a dreaded complication sometimes seen with long-term use of cuffed tracheostomy tubes. The continued pressure of an inflated cuff against the tracheal walls can impede circulation and lead to tissue damage. Trauma to tracheal tissue also occurs when rigid tracheostomy tubes are pulled out for changing. The tube scrapes against the back wall of the trachea on the way out, and when this is done frequently over a long period of time, severe damage can ensue. If one area of the trachea becomes irritated and suffers from ischemia, eventually the wall may erode away. Erosion can lead to hemorrhage or tracheo-esophageal fistula formation.

The first warnings of tracheal erosion may be persistent air leaks around an inflated cuff or the need to keep increasing the volume of air in the cuff to create an adequate seal. Fistula development may be detected by gastric contents being suctioned out through the tracheostomy when the cuff is deflated.

You can decrease the chances of tracheal erosion by several means. Make sure that tracheostomy tubes are removed carefully when they need to be changed. Try not to pull down on the tube too much as it comes out, since pulling out and down increases contact between the lower edge of the tube and the posterior tracheal wall. Encourage the use of the newer low-pressure pliable cuffs, that distribute low pressure evenly against the tracheal wall. High-pressure cuffs are more rigid and are usually those implicated in causing erosion.

SPECIALIZED AIDS TO RESPIRATION

The Rocking Bed

Some patients with neurologic dysfunction require assistance with lung ventilation, but their problems are not severe enough to warrant treatment with a respirator. These people may benefit from being placed on a rocking bed, if they are introduced to it gradually. With this bed, the body is tilted alternately from Trendelenburg to reverse Trendelenburg position. When the head is tilted up, the abdominal contents and diaphragm are lowered, making inspiration more effective. When the head is tilted downward, the abdominal contents push the diaphragm up into the chest and assist in expiration.

Electrophrenic Respiration

Spinal cord injury above C4 results in paralysis of the respiratory muscles, as mentioned before. People who survive such injuries are often destined to live the rest of their lives attached to a respirator. Recently, however, electrical stimulation of the phrenic nerve has been successfully performed, resulting in contraction of the diaphragm and therefore adequate ventilation without the use of a respirator. This new device has improved the quality of life for many quadriplegics.

Glossopharyngeal Breathing

This technique can be used by individuals who have continually shallow and monotonous respirations. It mimics the normal sign mechanism by pumping extra air into the lungs. The patient pulls in a mouthful and throatful of air, and by means of certain mouth and tongue movements, forces the air into the larynx and trachea. The motions are repeated rapidly until the lungs are fully inflated; then the patient exhales passively. Glossopharyngeal breathing, which is taught by respiratory therapists, can help to prevent atelectasis and hypostatic pneumonia.

NURSING MEASURES TO SUPPORT RESPIRATION IN NEUROLOGIC PATIENTS

There are many interventions a nurse can use to maximize ventilation and perfusion in neurologic patients whose respiratory function is affected. To know which interventions are appropriate, a definitive nursing assessment must first be done.

Assessment of Respiration

A good part of any respiratory assessment is done by means of inspection. Look at the patient's color, especially evaluating nail beds, extremities, and mucous membranes for cyanosis. Observe chest movements, watching to see which muscles are being used for inspiration, checking accessory muscles of the neck and shoulders in particular. When observing the chest, you should also look for symmetry of movement—whether both sides of the rib cage expand equally. Do the patient's respirations appear labored and difficult? Are there chest retractions? Is there any sighing? Is breathing a conscious effort rather than an unconscious process? Try to determine what the respiratory pattern is, as well as the rate. If you watch the patient during coughing, you can assess coughing force and effectiveness and observe sputum that is expectorated.

Asking the patient or family pertinent questions can give you some useful information. Find out if the patient is a smoker, and if so, how heavy a smoker. The possibility of chronic irritation from smoking may complicate the respiratory situation. Does the patient have a chronic cough or suffer from shortness of breath on exertion?

Auscultation of the chest is a necessary component of your assessment. Listen to breath sounds in all lobes routinely. In addition, auscultate before and after coughing or postural drainage to determine the effectiveness of these measures.

Check for the presence of gag and swallow reflexes by touching the back of the throat with an applicator or by stroking the throat. Ask the patient to swallow something, if possible, and watch the face and neck for asymmetry or muscle weakness. Table 5.1 contains a review of respiratory assessments and their significance.

Positioning

An unconscious patient with no artificial airway should be placed in the side-lying or semiprone position with the head of the bed flat to facilitate drainage of secretions. The neck should be slightly extended to prevent the tongue from blocking the pharynx. If the respirations become noisy or crowing in nature, the tongue may have slipped back against the pharyngeal wall. You can quickly remedy the situation by placing your fingers behind the angles of the mandible and pulling forward and upward, thus opening the airway.

The presence of a tracheostomy changes the situation slightly, since you do not have to worry about the tongue blocking the airway, but you do have to be concerned about positioning the patient so that the tracheostomy opening is not covered with bed linens.

TABLE 5.1 Respiratory Assessment

Parameter	Significance
Rate and rhythm	Watch for hypoventilation or hyperventilation. Assess pattern of respirations (see Chapter 1.) Should be periodic sighing.
Depth	Shallow respirations may indicate metabolic or muscular problems, and may lead to atelectasis.
Effort	Respiration should be effortless. Look for use of accessory muscles of neck and shoulders.
Sounds	Respiration should be silent. Auscultate for rales, wheezing, and rhonchi, which indicate increased or retained secretions. Listen for sounds of labored breathing.
Cough	Assess coughing force. Is cough productive or nonproductive? Does patient smoke?
Secretions	Assess color and thickness. Yellow or green sputum can indicate infection. Tenacious sputum may indicate need for more fluids.
Color (nail beds, mucous membranes, extremities)	Watch for cyanosis—a sign of hypoxemia.
Posture	Slumped position or poor posture can limit chest expansion and ventilation.
Chest movements	Asymmetry could indicate muscular paralysis or deformity. Chest retractions with depression of the sternum are seen mostly in children or thin adults who have labored respirations.

A conscious patient should have the head elevated to make the muscular work of respiration easier and to facilitate coughing. If the patient is capable of sitting in a chair, make sure that good posture is maintained. A weak patient naturally tends to slump down in the chair and hold the neck in slight flexion. Lung ventilation is compromised in such a position. Putting a small pillow in the lumbar area of the chair helps to prevent slouching and keeps the rib cage and chest in an upright position. Patients confined to bed should be repositioned frequently to prevent pooling of secretions in the lungs. The nursing care plan for your patient should have nursing orders that explain just how the patient should be positioned, where pillows are needed, and how often to change positions. Evaluate the plan frequently to make needed adjustments in care.

Postural Drainage

Manipulating a person's position to allow secretions to drain from the lungs by gravity is an old treatment, but one that is still very effective in helping the person with weak coughing force. Pillows are placed under the hips, back, stomach, or legs in order to raise various portions of the lungs and help them to drain. In many institutions, respiratory therapists are responsible for postural drainage, but the nurse may be involved in teaching the procedure to a patient who needs to continue doing it at home. For home treatment, most patients are simply taught to lie for 30 minutes on each side with a pillow under the hips.

Percussion (clapping) may also be done by a nurse or respiratory therapist, in conjunction with postural drainage. The chest wall is struck lightly and quickly with cupped hands, in the direction that you want the secretions to move. If it is desirable for percussion to be continued after discharge from the hospital, you can teach a family member the procedure.

Deep Breathing and Coughing

Neuromuscular disorders render a patient particularly susceptible to atelectasis, which means that you have to spend time assisting with deep breathing and coughing to promote lung inflation and remove secretions. Incentive spirometers or blow bottles have limited value for patients with weak respiratory muscles. Instead, you can use your hands on the patient's rib cage to apply pressure during expiration. This action prolongs expiration and leads to a deeper breath on the next inspiration. Repeat this procedure several times every 2 hours. The patient may eventually be able to assist with the external compression by wrapping the arms around the lower chest or upper abdomen and leaning forward on expiration.

Teaching a patient how to cough effectively in spite of weak muscles is another important nursing responsibility. Have the patient take a slow deep inhalation through the nose, then open the mouth and cough three times. As the patient reaches the peak of inspiration, apply pressure with your hands over the lower rib cage or upper abdomen (see Figure 5.5). The increase in pressure caused by your hands produces a high expiratory flow rate and can help to remove secretions.

Teaching effective coughing cannot usually be done in one session. You need to work with the patient over a period of time. Develop a teaching plan and record it in the card file (Kardex) for all nurses to

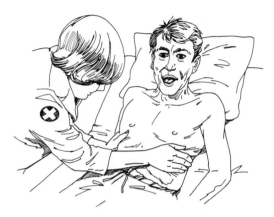

Figure 5.5 Manual pressure on the rib cage and upper abdomen at the end of inspiration helps to increase the force of coughing.

follow. Include specific nursing orders to guide the nurse who is teaching, such as "Instruct patient to take a slow deep breath through the nose, then cough with mouth open three times." After a few teaching sessions, evaluate how well the patient is coughing and using the information that has been given. You may have to revise your plan if you have not been successful.

It may be necessary for you to stimulate coughing in a patient who cannot follow commands or who cannot cough when requested to do so. One way to do this is to put finger pressure against the trachea near the cricoid cartilage. If external pressure does not work, you may have to insert a sterile suction catheter down into the trachea to trigger a cough. The patient with a tracheostomy may be forced to cough if 2 to 5 mℓ of saline is injected into the tracheostomy. If all these measures fail, suctioning alone may have to be relied on to remove secretions. The only time coughing should be discouraged is if there is a danger of or presence of increased intracranial pressure.

Adequate Hydration

Patients who are on oral intake should be encouraged to drink a lot of fluids. Fluids keep secretions thin and facilitate their removal during coughing. If oral fluids are not possible, parenteral fluid intake should be adequate to moisten secretions. In some patients, secretions remain tenacious in spite of fluid intake. Aerosol therapy may then be instituted by the physician. In this form of hydration, liquid particles are delivered directly into the airways by some type of nebulizer.

Cleaning of Nasal Passages

Comatose or paralyzed patients are prone to obstruction of the nares by dried secretions. This is one aspect of care that nurses give little thought to, yet the nasal passages serve a necessary function of warming and filtering inhaled air. Using a cotton-tipped applicator moistened with saline or diluted peroxide, gently moisten and remove secretions from the nose. After cleaning, apply a light layer of water-soluble lubricant to the mucous membranes with another applicator. If there is bleeding or cerebrospinal fluid leakage from the nose, consult the physician before cleaning the nares.

Teaching for Home Care

Planning for discharge of the neurologic patient with respiratory complications requires a lot of teaching and interdisciplinary referrals. In addition to teaching coughing or deep breathing or postural drainage procedures or use of nebulizers, patients may need to be taught self-tracheostomy care and suctioning. They must be taught the necessity of adequate hydration and good posture.

The patient's family is often included in teaching sessions if they are to be included in home care. Both patient and family need tremendous emotional support while learning and when coping with illness at home. They will probably require outside support systems such as a visiting nurse, a respiratory therapist, and perhaps a social worker. But for many patients and families, home care is infinitely preferable to hospitals and long-term-care facilities.

**EXAMPLES OF NURSING DIAGNOSES RELATED
TO ALTERED RESPIRATION**

Respiratory dysfunction related to retained secretions from failure to cough.

Respiratory dysfunction related to head injury; hypoventilation.

Respiratory dysfunction related to weakness of diaphragm and intercostal muscles.

Decreased cardiac output due to positive pressure of respirator.

Lack of comfort related to presence of tracheotomy tube.

Potential for hypoxia due to need for frequent suctioning.

Weak coughing force related to thoracic muscular weakness.

Tenacious secretions related to poor hydration.

Lack of knowledge related to postural drainage positions and procedure.

REFERENCES

Adams, Nancy R., "Prolonged Coma: Your Care Makes All the Difference," *Nursing 77*, 7, no. 8 (August 1977), p. 22.

Bushnell, Sharon Spaeth, *Respiratory Intensive Care Nursing*. Boston: Little, Brown and Company, 1973.

Ewertz, Marjorie, and Deborah Shpritz, "Your Best Strategy When 'Shock Lung' Strikes," *RN*, 43, no. 10 (October 1980), p. 43.

Hudak, Carolyn M., and others, *Critical Care Nursing*, 2nd ed. New York: J.B. Lippincott Company, 1977.

Kealy, Sandra L., "Respiratory Care in Guillain-Barré Syndrome," *American Journal of Nursing*, 77, no. 1 (January 1977), p. 58.

Lavigne, Jeanne M., "Respiratory Care of Patients with Neuromuscular Disease," *Nursing Clinics of North America*, 14, no. 1 (March 1979), p. 133.

Monahan, Colleen, and others, "Management of Ventilation following Spinal Cord Injury," *Respiratory Care*, 24, no. 11 (November 1979), p. 1011.

Nielson, Lois, "Mechanical Ventilation: Patient Assessment and Nursing Care," *American Journal of Nursing*, 80, no. 12 (December 1980), p. 2191.

Sykes, M.K., and others, *Respiratory Failure*, 2nd ed. Oxford: Blackwell Scientific Publications, 1976.

Walleck, Connie, "Pulmonary Complications in the Neurosurgical Patient," *Journal of Neurosurgical Nursing*, 9, no. 3 (September 1977), p. 102.

6

Alterations in Nutrition
and Fluid Balance

The unique nutritional and fluid problems that develop in the presence of neurologic disorders present a challenge for nurses. It is the nurse who monitors the patient's fluid balance most closely, and who evaluates the patient's appetite and food intake, and it is the nurse who is responsible for supplying needed nourishment. There are many independent nursing actions with which you should be familiar in order to maintain optimal nutritional status in your patients. But first you need an understanding of some of the ways in which nutrition and fluid balance are affected by neurologic problems.

NEUROLOGIC PATHOLOGY THAT AFFECTS
NUTRITION AND FLUID BALANCE

Cerebral Trauma

Immediately after a person has sustained a head injury, fluid and electrolyte balance begins to change. As in any stress state, antidiuretic hormone (ADH) is released in greater amounts than normal from the pituitary gland, and more aldosterone is produced by the adrenal glands. The resulting sodium and fluid retention is evident not only in laboratory tests results, but in decreased urinary output. When sodium is retained, potassium is excreted in abnormally large amounts, but the process usually reverses itself within a day or two, before the hypokalemia poses any great problem. Diuresis follows and fluids gradually return to normal unless there is continued fluid loss or other complications.

In some cerebral trauma cases, especially those involving skull fractures, damage to the pituitary or hypothalamus, or increased pressure in that area, may lead to *diabetes insipidus*. The hypothalamus may be unable to produce enough ADH, or the posterior pituitary may be unable to store the ADH, both problems leading to a decrease in ADH which normally acts on the kidneys to maintain water balance. In diabetes insipidus, then, too much water is excreted, leading to dehydration. The problem becomes evident when output greatly exceeds intake, and the patient complains of extreme thirst. Usually, this is a transitory dysfunction, but it may require medical treatment if fluid intake cannot keep up with output.

The same cerebral pathology sometimes leads to the exact opposite problem, in which too much ADH is secreted in excess of the body's need. The result is fluid retention and water intoxication. The patient may become very lethargic, confused, and eventually comatose. This sequence of events is termed the *syndrome of inappropriate ADH* (SIADH). If fluid restriction alone does not help to correct the problem, other medical intervention becomes necessary.

Nursing interventions.   Any patient who has sustained head trauma, whether from accident or surgery, should be kept on strict intake and output measurement. Very often urine output is measured hourly and fluid replacement is based on the amount of output. You must assess these measurements carefully, watching for trends such as continually increasing or decreasing urinary output.

Check the urine specific gravity every 4 hours, and if there is a noticeable change in output, check it every hour. Specific gravity is especially helpful in detecting diabetes insipidus because as output increases, the specific gravity continues to fall until it is almost the same as water, a measurement of 1.00. If you see abnormalities in fluid balance or urine concentration, report them to the physician immediately.

Even for a temporary case of diabetes insipidus, fluid intake must be increased and you will be responsible for regulating extra amounts of intravenous fluids, or if the patient is awake, of oral fluids. SIADH requires fluid restriction, so you will have to make sure that the patient adheres to oral fluid restriction, or that intravenous fluids are kept to the ordered limit. If the patient is alert, your explanations and support can make these necessary fluid changes more acceptable and less burdensome to the patient.

A severe change in fluid balance due to ADH disturbance may necessitate the use of drug therapy. Diabetes insipidus is treated with injectable pitressin for short-term therapy, or with nasal spray solutions such as desmopressin (DDAVP) for long-term therapy. Very mild cases may be controlled with the oral hypoglycemic agent chlorpropamide (Diabenese), which enhances the release and use of ADH. SIADH may respond to administration of furosemide (Lasix), a potent diuretic, or demeclocycline hydrochloride (Declomycin), an antibiotic that blocks the effect of ADH on the kidney. Even though drug therapy is initiated, you must still assess intake and output carefully until the patient is stabilized on the drug.

General Central Nervous System Trauma

The person who becomes critically ill as a result of severe trauma anywhere in the central nervous system (CNS) is subject to disturbances in the functioning of the gastrointestinal tract. Stress ulcers, gastric dilation, or paralytic ileus can all occur.

Stress ulcers associated with CNS trauma are termed *Cushing's ulcers*. They are thought to occur following an episode of shock in which there is a decrease in blood flow to the gastric mucosa. At the same time, stress precipitates an increase in gastric acidity and an increase in steroid levels, all of which lead to a breakdown in the gastric mucosa. Cushing's ulcers are often very deep and penetrating, prone to hemorrhage, and swift to develop.

Gastric dilatation occurs in some critically ill patients who have artificial airways in place. The irritation of the airway causes excessive swallowing, and a large amount of air enters the stomach. Lack of peristalsis also contributes to gastric distention because gastric secretions remain pooled in the stomach. A distended stomach is uncomfortable and can interfere with ventilation as well as predisposing to vomiting and aspiration.

CNS trauma, whether to the brain or spinal cord, can affect autonomic control of bowel function, with paralytic ileus resulting. Unless treatment is instituted, massive amounts of fluid and electrolytes can move into the intestines, dehydrating body tissues and sometimes ending in hypovolemic shock.

Nursing implications. Stress ulcers can be prevented in many patients by giving antacids via nasogastric tube and cimetidine (Tagamet) intravenously during the period of critical illness. Tagamet inhibits the action of histamine in the stomach and thus reduces gastric acid secretion. Throughout this time your observations of nasogastric drainage and stool are very important. Watch especially for hematemesis or melena, which result from severe gastric erosion or perforation. Also observe whether stools are too hard or too soft. Antacids whose primary ingredient is aluminum tend to be constipating. Those whose major ingredient is magnesium may cause diarrhea.

Assess the patient's bowel sounds and abdominal girth to detect early signs of paralytic ileus or gastric distention. If a nasogastric tube or intestinal tube is in place, check the patency of the tube routinely and monitor output from it. The physician may order fluid replacement for the amount of intestinal or gastric fluid removed each shift, so exact measurement is essential.

Changes in Oral Sensation

The condition having the most devastating effects on oral sensation is *trigeminal neuralgia.* Occurring in later adulthood and of unknown cause, trigeminal neuralgia consists of severe paroxysms of pain in one side of the face along one or more branches of the trigeminal nerve. Episodes of pain may be triggered by touching the face, teeth, or tongue, or by exposure to a cold breeze or by foods of extreme temperatures.

Eating becomes a real source of distress because it invokes the fear of pain or sets off an attack of pain. The most successful treatments for trigeminal neuralgia have been alcohol injections into the nerve branches, or surgical destruction of various portions of the nerve. In either case, one of the troublesome residual effects of such therapy is temporary or permanent anesthesia in the area supplied by the treated nerve.

Nursing management.   Preoperatively, patients suffering from this distressing problem should be helped to find ways to avoid pain. You can assist the patient to choose semisolid or liquid foods which are nourishing. Check the temperature of the food before giving it to the patient; extremes of temperature must be avoided. Chewing the food on the uninvolved side of the mouth may also help to limit pain.

Postoperatively, some of the same precautions must be observed, but for different reasons. If there is anesthesia of the mucous membranes of the mouth, there is also the danger of injury to those areas, of which the patient would not be aware. You should instruct the person to chew food on the side that has sensation and to eat foods of moderate temperatures. The patient must inspect the affected side of the mouth frequently to look for possible damage that may have resulted from biting the cheek or burning the mucous membranes. Good mouth care is essential to prevent oral complications.

Paralysis of Muscles of Chewing or Swallowing

Neurologic basis of swallowing.   The act of swallowing is very complex, involving many motor neurons, cranial nerves, and muscles. The cranial nerves controlling the sensations that trigger the swallowing reflex are the trigeminal, glossopharyngeal, and vagus. They convey the stimulus to the medulla, where the complex sequence of inhibiting respiration and permitting swallowing at the same time is controlled.

The cranial nerves that are involved in the motor aspects of swallowing are the trigeminal, facial, glossopharyngeal, vagus, and hypoglossal. The muscles of the tongue, palate, pharynx, larynx, and esophagus are innervated by these cranial nerves, together with various motor neurons in the cervical spinal cord.

Swallowing takes place in the following manner. After food or fluid has been placed in the mouth, the tongue, under voluntary control, pushes it back and up against the soft palate and keeps it there while the larynx is pulled upward under the epiglottis to close the airway. At the same time, the soft palate is elevated and blocks off the nasopharynx to prevent food from entering the nasal cavity. Once the airway and nose have been occluded, the bolus of food moves into the pharynx and is propelled into the esophagus, where peristaltic waves carry it to the stomach.

There are many physiologic dysfunctions of the nervous system which in some way impair the swallowing reflex and the muscle movements of chewing. The most common problems will be mentioned.

Hemiplegia. Paralysis of the muscles of one side of the face and throat can cause serious difficulties in chewing and swallowing. Such paralysis may result from damage to the motor neurons or cranial nerves that innervate the muscles. The gag reflex may be diminished or absent, the swallowing reflex may be affected, and the voluntary muscular actions of sucking, chewing, and swallowing may be impaired. If food is placed in the mouth, it may be pocketed in the cheeks, aspirated, or it may just fall out of the mouth. These types of problems are often seen in patients with a stroke, Bell's palsy, or bulbar palsy.

Cerebral Palsy. The child or adult with cerebral palsy may present unique feeding problems. As in the case of hemiplegia, there may be difficulty with sucking and chewing. But the most difficult problem to overcome is tongue thrusting or reversal of the wavelike movements that normally propel food to the back of the mouth. Although this situation is seen most commonly in cerebral palsy, it may sometimes occur in stroke patients as well.

Nursing interventions. The individual who has dysphagia and related disorders can suffer from severe nutritional problems. It often takes so long to feed these patients that it seems as if you are simply moving from one meal to the next. Other nursing activities are also demanding your time, and as a result, you may stop feeding a patient before all necessary nutrients have been given or before the patient's appetite is assuaged. If this pattern continues, the patient will lose weight and suffer nutritional deficiencies.

It may seem impossible to get food into the patient. You will have to use new techniques to feed a patient whose tongue gets in the way or who does not swallow by reflex. If regular feeding methods become dangerous because the gag reflex is not operating normally, you will have to use a different method of supplying nutrients, such as tube feedings.

Testing Gag and Swallowing Reflexes.   Before attempting to feed a patient who has suffered neurologic damage, you must test for gag and swallowing reflexes. Depressing the tongue with a tongue blade and then touching the back of the throat with a cotton-tipped applicator should evoke the gag response and perhaps also stimulate swallowing. If the gag reflex is weak, feeding should be done with care. If it is absent, food and fluids should be withheld.

A more specific test of swallowing involves putting a small amount of a semisolid food in the patient's mouth. You will find that foods such as ice cream, custard, or farina are good for this purpose. They are solid enough to stimulate the swallowing reflex, yet not as apt to be aspirated as a thin fluid. Suction equipment should be at hand in case the patient does begin to aspirate.

Chewing involves a different set of abilities and muscular function and should be tested with soft foods such as bread or cheese. You can still supply a nutritious diet even if the muscles of chewing are weak. Meats, for example, can be chopped or pureed for someone who has difficulty chewing.

Feeding the Patient with Dysphagia.   Positioning your patient previous to mealtimes is an important step in the feeding process. Try to position the patient about 15 to 30 minutes before feeding to let the patient get settled and prepared to eat. If a sitting position is possible, provide for adequate support with pillows to prevent leaning. You can prevent the patient's sliding down in the chair by placing a small rolled towel under the knee area (for short time periods only, to prevent impairment of circulation). A patient without head control should be placed in a semi-Fowler's position in bed, or else you can hold the head up by placing your hand on the patient's forehead. A hemiplegic patient who cannot sit should be turned on the unaffected side for meals, so that food will stay on the unimpaired side of the mouth.

Patients who do not open their lips voluntarily in response to the sight of food or to your request can often be stimulated to do so (see Figure 6.1). Do not try to force the mouth open, but instead just gently touch the spoon to the lips. If this approach does not work, try placing

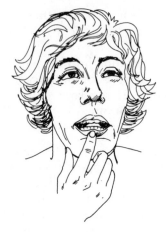

Figure 6.1 Opening the patient's lips.

your finger on the chin directly beneath the lower lip and apply light pressure. Do this several times, without force, and the mouth will probably open.

Food placement is an important consideration in feeding hemiplegic patients and those who have tongue thrusting. For hemiplegic patients, place the food on the functioning side of the mouth, where it can be felt and manipulated. In the case of tongue protrusion, food should be placed toward the back of the tongue, making it less likely to be expelled from the mouth. If this last approach does not work, or if you cannot get the food past the tongue, try applying pressure under the mandible; this pressure may bring the tongue back into the mouth.

Next, the patient may need help in closing the lips (see Figure 6.2). You can place one finger above the upper lip and apply pressure, or gently pinch both lips together between your fingers. Sometimes just stroking the lips with your finger may be enough to stimulate closing.

Once the lips are closed, your next concern is swallowing. Several techniques may be useful in initiating swallowing. Start with telling the

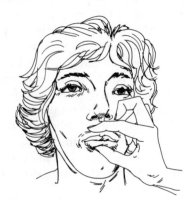

Figure 6.2 Holding the lips closed.

patient to swallow; a reminder may be all that is needed. If that is not successful, try stroking the throat, moving one finger gently down the midline of the larynx. Allowing the patient to smell the food may also help to encourage swallowing. Keep the patient's head flexed slightly forward at this point. This position makes swallowing easier and makes aspiration less likely since the esophagus is wide open and the airway is narrowed. After you have observed the swallow, look in the mouth to make sure that all food is gone before giving another spoonful.

Brain-damaged patients who are capable of chewing may forget to do so. You can simply remind them to chew when necessary, and can manipulate the jaw up and down to start them off with the right action. If drooling occurs, tell the patient about it and encourage licking the lips to prevent dripping. Wiping the patient's face when necessary will also bring about awareness of drooling.

Implements that can be used in feeding dysphagic patients include a spoon, cup, straw, or syringe. A spoon should always be used rather than a fork, which can cause injury. Spoon feeding of liquids can be very tedious, so use of a plastic cup or straw is preferable. If the patient cannot suck, a straw may not be feasible, but it may be possible to use the straw by placing it in the fluid, putting your finger over the top opening, and then inserting the bottom end of the straw into the mouth and releasing your finger, allowing the fluid to run into the mouth (see Figure 6.3). The advantage to using a plastic cup is that larger amounts of fluid can be given, which in some cases helps to stimulate swallowing.

A bulb syringe is useful in delivering fluids to a patient with a protruding tongue. The tapered syringe end can slide over the tongue and place the fluid toward the back of the mouth. You must be careful, though, not to push in too much liquid at one time, and not to push air into the mouth. Piston (barrel and plunger) syringes should be avoided

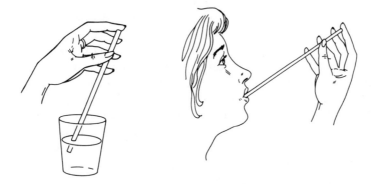

Figure 6.3 Trapping fluid in the straw and then releasing it into the patient's mouth.

for this purpose because it is difficult to control the amount and rate of fluid being pushed into the mouth.

Some cases of dysphagia are very difficult to deal with and you may not be successful with the approaches described above. Give each approach a few trials to ascertain whether it will work with your patient. If you find that the approach you are using is not helping the patient to chew or swallow, and intake is not improving, try another method. If after several trials and evaluations you still are not solving the problem, contact a physical therapist, occupational therapist, or speech pathologist. Any of these specialists may be able to help assess and treat the problem.

When a successful method of feeding the dysphagic patient has been established, write detailed nursing orders in the patient's care plan which explain exactly how to proceed. An explicit plan will eliminate the need for each nurse to use trial-and-error methods.

Feeding the Patient with a Tracheostomy.   Oral feedings should be given with great care in the presence of a tracheostomy. Tracheostomy tubes may interfere with swallowing by anchoring the trachea and preventing the larynx from moving up and closing the airway. Large tubes (over size 5) and cuffed tubes may also impinge on the esophagus. Both of these factors increase the incidence of aspiration of oral feedings. Even if a cuff is inflated, liquids or solid food may be aspirated and rest on top of the cuff. The force of swallowing may push some of the food around the cuff into the airways.

Tube Feedings.   Supplying nourishment through a nasogastric tube is one of the preferred feeding methods in patients who cannot swallow. Tube feedings are relatively easy to do and are associated with fewer complications than intravenous therapy. Adequate nutrients can be given for a long period of time if certain precautions are maintained.

The solution being administered is ordered by the physician. The options are blenderized hospital food in specific proportions of fat, carbohydrates, and protein, or commercially prepared formulas such as Ensure or Vivonex. Hospital-prepared feedings must be kept refrigerated and then warmed before administration, to prevent cramping and diarrhea. Commercial formulas can be stored at room temperature.

The feeding may be administered intermittently, such as 200 mℓ every 4 hours, or continuously by slow drip. The intermittent method is preferable unless the patient can be monitored by a nurse almost constantly. Aspiration of stomach contents is more likely to happen with continuous feedings.

When giving a tube feeding, you must be aware of some critical nursing measures. The head of the bed must be elevated 40 to 60 degrees throughout the feeding and for at least 30 minutes afterward. If the feeding is continuous, the head must be elevated continuously. This may best be accomplished by putting the bed in reverse Trendelenburg position, thus making it still possible to turn the patient from side to side. Correct positioning reduces the incidence of aspiration. A nursing order stating, "Elevate the head of the bed 40 to 60 degrees during and for 30 minutes after feeding" must be written on the care plan.

It is also essential to aspirate the stomach contents before each intermittent feeding. This not only assures you that the tube is in the stomach, but it allows you to assess how well the patient is digesting the previous feeding. If more than 80 to 100 mℓ of fluid remains in the stomach, tell the physician so that new orders can be written. Whatever residual amount remains and is removed from the stomach must be returned to it, since it contains needed gastric acids. But you must subtract the amount of residual from the amount of fluid to be given in the next feeding. For example, you plan to administer 200 mℓ of formula with 50 mℓ of water after the feeding. If the stomach residual is 80 mℓ, you will put it back into the stomach and only give 120 mℓ of formula with 50 mℓ of water.

There are a few problems associated with tube feedings. The first and most dangerous is aspiration. As already mentioned, the chances of aspiration can be minimized by positioning the patient correctly, by not overfilling the stomach, and by staying with the patient during feedings. In addition, you should add food coloring to white or beige formulas so that you can recognize feedings that might have been aspirated and are later coughed up or suctioned from the bronchial tree.

Diarrhea is a frequent problem that may result from cold feedings or from formulas high in carbohydrates, fats, or proteins. Concentrated solutions produce a hyperosmolar state in the intestines, which causes water to move into the area, leading to diarrhea. You can help to prevent the problem by warming formulas that have been refrigerated and by giving extra water between feedings. Water helps to reduce the hyperosmolarity and to supply the patient with needed hydration.

Dehydration can occur if the individual has prolonged diarrhea, and also if the formula feedings are the patient's only intake. A relatively small amount of fluid is given in most tube feedings, perhaps only 1500 to 1800 mℓ per day. Therefore, giving water between feedings will not only help to prevent diarrhea, but it will protect the patient against dehydration from diarrhea and low intake.

Enteral Hyperalimentation.   This feeding method is similar to the older standard tube feedings in that a formula is infused through a nasogastric tube, and many of the same problems can develop. Enteral hyperalimentation, though, is always done by continuous drip and can be used to deliver high concentrations of nutrients and calories. Commercially prepared solutions such as Vivonex HN, Ensure Plus, and Amin-Aid provide as many as 1500 kilocalories (kcal) per 1,000 ml because of the large amount of carbohydrates, and contain high concentrations of protein for wound healing. They are useful in the treatment of very malnourished and underweight patients, perhaps patients who have been maintained on intravenous fluids or regular tube feedings for a long time.

In order to prevent metabolic disturbances from such hyperosmolar solutions, the formulas are usually started at half strength and gradually increased to full strength over a few days. After a week or so, it is possible to give the patient as many as 4000 to 5000 kcal per day.

Inevitably, such a concentrated mixture causes some problems. Diarrhea is the most common symptom, which can be controlled by slowing down the solution, or if that is not advisable, by administering antidiarrheals. Glucosuria is a possibility because of the large carbohydrate load. Urine sugar and acetone levels should be checked every 4 to 6 hours. If the patient begins to spill sugar, insulin may be given. The patient's weight should be checked every day or two to determine the effectiveness of treatment. Nursing orders must be written to cover these procedures. For example, one order might state, "Urine S&A Q4H and report *any* glucosuria." Another might read, "Weigh OD at 7:30 a.m. only in pajamas, record, and report changes of more than 1 pound."

Gastrostomy Feedings. When it becomes apparent that a dysphagic patient will not be able to return to oral feedings, a gastrostomy tube may have to be inserted. Nasogastric tube feedings cannot be used indefinitely because of irritation and possible necrosis of the esophagus. Intravenous therapy does not supply all the nutrients necessary to support life for a long period of time and is associated with many complications. That leaves the gastrostomy tube as the best long-term alternative. A small incision is made into the stomach under local anesthesia, and the tube is inserted and sutured in place.

The same procedure is used to administer a gastrostomy tube feeding as is used for nasogastric tube feedings. Precautions should be taken in the first few days to prevent infection at the insertion site. You must keep the skin free of gastric secretions that can cause maceration.

Mouth Care. This routine aspect of nursing care is of utmost importance for all dysphagic patients, those who are on oral feedings, and especially those who are NPO or are receiving tube feedings. A patient who is on oral feedings may not be swallowing all the food in the mouth. Also, this person may not be capable of moving the tongue around to clean the teeth. So after each feeding you have to inspect the mouth and give mouth care to prevent tooth and gum problems or general stomatitis.

Those patients who are NPO are susceptible to *parotitis*, inflammation of the salivary glands. Poor oral hygiene makes the person even more prone to this disorder. Oral suctioning may also add to the risk by introducing more bacteria to the area. If you pay special attention to mouth care, emphasizing it in your nursing orders, you may avoid such problems.

If there is swallowing ability and the patient is fairly alert, mouth care may simply consist of brushing the teeth and tongue and rinsing them. However, if there is no swallowing capability, you have to be concerned about aspiration. You may brush the teeth, but rinsing becomes a problem. You can try irrigating the mouth with a syringe while the patient is lying on one side, letting some of the water run out of the mouth, and suctioning out any that is in the back of the mouth. This procedure may require two people, one to irrigate and the other to suction. If you think that there is still a risk of aspiration, perhaps because of difficulty in positioning the patient, you may have to resort to an alternative procedure.

A padded tongue depressor soaked in peroxide and water or mouthwash can be used to wipe off the teeth, tongue, and gums. In some cases, this is all you can do. Glycerine can then be used to keep the mucous membranes soft and prevent irritation. The lips may also need a glycerine coating to prevent cracking. If you have difficulty getting into the mouth because the patient bites down, try to get the mouth open for at least a few seconds so that you can insert a bite block, which will hold the teeth open while you clean the mouth. Some patients just cannot open their mouths, and you will only be able to clean the exterior portion of the teeth and gums.

NUTRITIONAL AND FLUID NEEDS
OF THE NEUROLOGIC PATIENT

The neurologic patient may be chronically or acutely ill, and in either case may have special nutritional and fluid needs. These needs are frequently neglected by some physicians and nurses, who do not stop to calculate nutritional needs or who believe that for short-term illness no special treatment is necessary.

Caloric and Nutritional Requirements

Anyone who is in a stressed state needs extra calories and protein and perhaps replacement of certain vitamins or minerals. A stressed state can be severe trauma, fever, surgery, or even continuous tremors or athetoid movements. All of these situations call for more energy to meet metabolic needs. If extra nutrients are not supplied, the individual will go into a catabolic state, in which fat and protein will be broken down for energy. A negative nitrogen balance will develop, indicating that more nitrogen is being used than is being taken into the body.

How does this nutritional catastrophe happen? In many cases, acutely ill or traumatized patients are maintained only on intravenous therapy until the condition is stabilized. Days go by in which the patient is literally being starved. Being on bedrest contributes to the problem, since inactive tissue breaks down at a fast rate. Even if the patient can eat, many tests may be ordered that require the patient to be NPO. Tube feedings may be started, but too often they are given in insufficient amounts or their composition is nutritionally inadequate.

The end result of such starvation is malnutrition. There is rapid weight loss, weakness, muscle wasting, poor wound healing, increased susceptibility to infection, edema, and anemia. If you add all these effects to the effects of the initial disease or injury, a very serious situation develops.

But hospital-induced malnutrition can be prevented. You should evaluate the situation, the patient's needs, and the nourishment that is being given. If the patient is beginning to show signs of malnutrition, or you think it is likely to develop, bring it to the physician's attention and perhaps suggest some alternatives. Because you spend a lot of time with a patient, you may know best how to supply needed nutrients.

The patient who is able to swallow may need between-meal nutritional supplements that are high in calories and protein. The dysphagic patient may require supplemental tube feedings or enteral hyperalimentation. The patient who cannot tolerate any type of feeding because of a nonfunctioning gastrointestinal tract may need parenteral hyperalimentation.

A normal person at rest requires about 1000 to 1500 kcal to maintain normal weight and good nutritional balance. An ill person whose body is trying to repair itself, or who is restless, or who has even a low-grade fever, may need double or triple the calories, even though the body is presumably still at rest.

Fluid Requirements

Most patients in stressed states also require increased amounts of fluids. Fluid may be lost through open wounds, diarrhea, hyperventilation, or fever. It may also be trapped in a space where it cannot be used. Decreased fluid intake results in dehydration and inadequate urinary output.

The combination of inactivity and dehydration can lead to serious urinary tract problems. Stasis of urine in the kidneys and bladder, together with a decreased flow or urine from low output, can predispose the patient to urinary infection. Renal calculi may form because of low output and excretion of calcium which has been lost from the bones.

You can help prevent dehydration and urinary problems. Keep strict intake and output records. Maintain a good oral intake when possible by offering the patient's favorite fluids at frequent intervals, and write a nursing order specifying which fluids are preferred and how much should be given and when. Give extra water to tube-fed patients, and make sure that you keep intravenous fluids on time. You can spare the patient many problems if you monitor fluids closely and maintain a 3000 mℓ intake, unless contraindicated.

Parenteral Therapy

The person who cannot take adequate fluids by mouth may need parenteral fluid therapy. Intravenous therapy is commonly used for the acutely or critically ill patient to supply needed fluids and electrolytes. For long-term therapy, the patient who cannot tolerate food or fluids in the gastrointestinal tract may require parenteral hyperalimentation.

Intravenous therapy.   Standard intravenous therapy is invaluable in helping to restore acutely ill patients to fluid and electrolyte balance. The major drawback to this type of fluid replacement or maintenance is that no protein and not enough calories are supplied in order to prevent protein-calorie malnutrition. One frequently used maintenance solution, 1000 mℓ of 5% dextrose and water, contains only about 170 kcal. If 3000 mℓ is given per day, the patient receives about 510 kcal, not nearly enough even to meet the body's minimum needs.

Other disadvantages of intravenous therapy include the necessity to change insertion sites every 2 to 3 days, the danger of infection, thrombophlebitis, and infiltration. Your aseptic technique must be impeccable in handling intravenous (IV) equipment. Strict routines should be followed in regard to changing tubing every 24 to 48 hours and giving IV site care every day. Evaluate the effectiveness of IV care for your patient. If complications are occurring, more attention must be given to this aspect of care. With careful technique, complications can be reduced.

After oral feedings are begun, IV therapy may continue to be used to supply a patient with additional fluids, electrolytes, and perhaps intravenous medications. As long as standard IVs are not the patient's only source of nutrition, they can continue to play a valuable supportive role.

Parenteral hyperalimentation.   Also known as *total parenteral nutrition*

(TPN), this form of intravenous therapy is used for long-term therapy to supply needed calories and protein, thus maintaining nitrogen balance and body weight.

Hyperalimentation solution contains high concentrations of dextrose (20 to 50%) to supply calories, amino acids as a protein nitrogen source, vitamins, electrolytes, and trace minerals. Most solutions provide about 1000 kcal per liter. It is therefore possible to meet all the patient's nutritional needs parenterally.

Because the solutions are hypertonic, they usually cannot be delivered into a peripheral vein; the high concentration of ingredients leads to phlebitis and thrombosis. Instead, a catheter is placed in the right or left subclavian or jugular veins and threaded into the superior vena cava. In the vena cava, blood flow is great enough to dilute quickly the hypertonic solution.

Calories and essential fatty acids can be supplied by newer solutions called *fat emulsions*. These solutions supply even more concentrated calories but in an isotonic solution, so a peripheral vein can be used.

Nursing responsibilities in caring for a patient receiving hyperalimentation are quite extensive. Maintaining the exact flow rate of the

TABLE 6.1 Assessment of Nutritional and Fluid Balance

Parameter	Significance
Body weight	A 1-pound gain or loss may reflect retention or excretion of 500 ml of fluid. Gains or losses may also indicate need for diet change.
24-hour intake and output	If intake is vastly greater than output, fluid retention may exist. If output is greater than intake, the patient may have diabetes insipidus or a hyperosmolar state (perhaps from hyperalimentation).
24-hour calorie count	May indicate need for nutritional supplements or dietary restrictions.
Skin condition	Poor skin turgor and dry skin may indicate dehydration. Delayed wound healing can be due to protein depletion.
Tongue and mucous membrane condition	Sticky mucous membranes may result from dehydration and electrolyte imbalance.
Vein filling	Delayed vein filling indicates decreased fluid volume in intravascular compartment.
Temperature	Slight elevations are often seen in dehydration.
Mental status	Agitation and confusion may result from severe fluid depletion. Decreased level of consciousness occurs with water intoxication.

fluid is crucial; for this reason an infusion pump is often used. If the solution infuses too slowly, you are depriving the patient of needed nutrients. If it runs in too fast, there is danger to the fluid and glucose balance of the body because of the hypertonicity of the solution.

Sugar and acetone measurements must be taken every 6 hours to determine whether the sugar load is too great for the body to handle. The patient may be placed on insulin coverage. Intake and output records will help you to see whether osmotic diuresis is taking place. The patient is weighed every day to determine the effectiveness of treatment. Most patients gain weight while on hyperalimentation.

Caution is used in all aspects of the treatment to make sure that contamination does not occur, because septicemia is a possibility when a catheter is placed in a major blood vessel and kept there for relatively long periods of time. Dressing changes are done three times a week with strict sterile technique, sometimes by one nurse who is assigned to do all hyperalimentation dressings in the hospital. To decrease the chance of bacterial growth in the IV tubing, change it each time you hang a new bottle. The concentrated dextrose in the tubing is an excellent culture medium for bacteria. No other medications or solutions may be added to the hyperalimentation line. Additives increase the chance of contamination and may not be compatible.

Assessment of Nutritional and Fluid Balance

You should do periodic assessments of nutritional status and fluid balance on any neurologic patient whose oral intake is questionable or who is receiving nutritional or fluid therapy. Following are the components of the assessment (see also Table 6.1).

Body weight.   Weigh the patient at the same time each day, with the patient wearing the same clothing. Weight fluctuations can result from tissue gains or losses or from fluid retention or loss. Very rapid weight gain or loss is more likely to be due to a change in fluid status. It is estimated that retention or excretion of 500 mℓ of fluid will alter the patient's weight by 1 pound.

24-Hour intake and output.   Measuring the patient's fluid intake and output and comparing them for a 24-hour period will give you an idea of whether fluid is being retained or whether diuresis is occurring for some reason. Remember that urine output will normally be less than intake due to insensible water loss through respiration, perspiration, and stools.

24-Hour calorie count.   This assessment is usually done in cooperation with a dietitian. Nurses record all foods in approximate amounts that the patient eats in 24 hours. The dietitian then calculates the number of calories that were eaten. This may be done for several days in a row. The information gained may be used in several ways. A low caloric intake may indicate the need for nutritional supplements. High intake may also show the need for a diet change or reduction. Adequate intake in the presence of weight loss may indicate that there is a different cause for the weight loss other than poor nutrition. Calorie counts in conjunction with 24-hour urine collection can be used to determine nitrogen balance.

Skin condition.   Changes in skin condition may occur with either nutritional deficits or fluid imbalance. A patient very prone to skin breakdown and who has poor wound healing may be suffering from protein depletion. Poor skin turgor is a sign of dehydration. You can easily check skin turgor by gently pinching up some skin over the clavicle. When released, normal skin will immediately flatten out. Dehydrated skin may remain pinched up for several seconds.

Edema in the tissues under the skin can result from lack of protein intake with consequent decreased plasma proteins. Plasma proteins hold fluid in the intravascular space. If they are decreased, fluid is lost to the interstitial spaces, and may settle in dependent portions of the body such as the ankles or sacral area.

Tongue and mucous membrane condition.   If you look at normal mucous membranes, you will see that they are shiny from moisture. Fluid loss may cause mucous membranes to be sticky and appear dry and dull. The tongue may also become sticky and furrowed. When the mouth becomes this dry, the patient may complain of thirst, another sign of dehydration.

Vein filling.   Hold your patient's hand at heart level and occlude the distal end of a small vein. Then stroke it toward the heart to empty it. When you take your finger off the distal end, the vein should fill immediately. Very slow filling tells you that there is decreased fluid volume in the body.

Temperature.   A slightly elevated body temperature can indicate dehydration. Body fluid is needed to conduct heat to the outside of the body. If there is not enough fluid to do this, the temperature may go up. Other possible causes of an elevated temperature should also be ruled out.

Mental status.   A patient with severe fluid depletion may exhibit unusual behavior, such as agitation, confusion, and disorientation. A change in level of consciousness, such as lethargy, may also result. Water intoxication caused by severe fluid retention can also cause a decrease in level of consciousness.

Anthropometric measurements. Measuring skinfold thicknesses and muscle size can give an indication of whether body fat and muscle mass has been depleted due to poor nutrition. Usually, the physician orders this kind of assessment and the dietitian does it, sometimes with the assistance of the nurse.

Laboratory tests. Although the physician orders lab tests and evaluates the results, you can also check the lab slips to help gain information for your assessment. Dehydration leads to an increase in hematocrit, blood urea nitrogen (BUN), and urine specific gravity. Protein malnutrition may be indicated by decreased serum albumin and urinary creatinine.

If you have questions about a patient's nutritional status or are unsure about the significance of your assessment findings, consult the patient's dietitian, who may be able to supply you with more information and expert advice. Use any resources you need in your planning and interventions to meet your patient's nutritional needs. Nutrition is a very important determinant of the patient's recovery and continued health.

**EXAMPLES OF NURSING DIAGNOSES RELATED
TO ALTERATIONS IN NUTRITION AND FLUID BALANCE**

Fluid retention related to stress state; dependent edema and low urine output.

Fluid volume deficit related to temporary diabetes insipidus.

Discomfort related to Cushing's ulcer.

Alteration in nutrition related to hemiplegia with impaired swallowing.

Potential for injury to oral mucosa due to lack of oral sensation.

Difficulty taking in food related to tongue thrusting.

Potential for aspiration related to weak gag reflex.

Weight loss related to feeding difficulties and refusal of food.

Diarrhea related to tube feedings.

Potential for stomatitis or parotitis related to lack of intake and difficulty opening mouth.

Altered self-concept related to inability to feed self.

Dehydration related to poor intake.

REFERENCES

Adams, Nancy R., "Prolonged Coma; Your Care Makes All the Difference," *Nursing 77*, 7, no. 8 (August 1977), p. 22.

Anderson, Barbara Jo, "Antidiuretic Hormone: Balance and Imbalance," *Journal of Neurosurgical Nursing*, 11, no. 2 (June 1979), p. 71.

Borgen, Linda, "Total Parenteral Nutrition in Adults," *American Journal of Nursing*, 78, no. 2 (February 1978), p. 224.

Buckley, John E., and others, "Feeding Patients with Dysphagia," *Nursing Forum*, 15, no. 1 (January 1976), p. 69.

Coyle, Nessa, and Ehud Arbit, "How to Protect Your Patients against Aspiration Pneumonia," *Nursing 78*, 8, no. 10 (October 1978), p. 50.

Demi-Resnick, Patty, "Unscrambling the Dietician's Report," *RN*, 44, no. 7 (July 1981), p. 52.

Donovan, Lynn, "Is the Doctor Starving Your Patient?", *RN*, 41, no. 7 (July 1978), p. 36.

Gaffney, Terry Weiler, and Rosemary Peterson Campbell, "Feeding Techniques for Dysphagic Patients," *American Journal of Nursing*, 74, no. 12 (December 1974), p. 2194.

Glaser, Suzanne, "How to Improve the First Stage of Digestion," *Geriatric Nursing*, 2, no. 5 (September–October 1981), p. 350.

Green, Marilyn, and Joann Harry, *Nutrition in Contemporary Nursing Practice*. New York: John Wiley & Sons, Inc., 1981.

Griggs, Barbara A., and Mary C. Hoppe, "Update: Nasogastric Tube Feeding," *American Journal of Nursing*, 79, no. 3 (March 1979), p. 481.

Guzman, Lani, "Don't Forget 'Nursing' When You're in the ICU," *RN*, 43, no. 12 (December 1980), p. 1B.

Kubo, Winifred, and others, "Fluid and Electrolyte Problems of Tube-Fed Patients," *American Journal of Nursing*, 76, no. 6 (June 1976), p. 912.

Persons, Carol, "Why Risk TPN When Tube Feeding Will Do," *RN*, 44, no. 1 (January 1981), p. 35.

Salmond, Susan Warner, "How to Assess the Nutritional Status of Acutely Ill Patients," *American Journal of Nursing*, 80, no. 5 (May 1980), p. 922.

Treharne, Dilys A., "Management of Feeding Difficulties," *Nursing Times*, 75, no. 3 (January 18, 1979), p. 108.

7

Alterations in Communication

A person who has a language deficit or who does not communicate in a normal way faces tremendous practical and emotional problems, because the defect cannot be hidden and because it interferes with interpersonal relationships and the satisfaction of human needs. Whether the problem is the total inability to use language as a means of communicating, or whether the problem is slurred speech or difficulty in reading, everyday life is affected, and the person needs help. The nurse has a very definite role in helping people with communication problems, just as the speech pathologist or therapist does. The ways in which the nurse can assist with these problems are explained in this chapter.

LANGUAGE ALTERATIONS DUE TO STROKE OR BRAIN TRAUMA

The areas of the brain that contain language centers can be damaged by lack of blood supply or by trauma to brain tissue. Stroke often results in necrosis of one or more language areas or the fibers connecting them. Trauma from automobile accidents, gunshot wounds, or tumor growth can damage the brain tissues that control language.

Wernicke's area (see Figure 7.1) is found in the temporal lobe and functions to make sense of incoming communication and to sort out messages that are to be expressed in return. Broca's area is located in the frontal lobe near the motor cortex and is primarily responsible for the

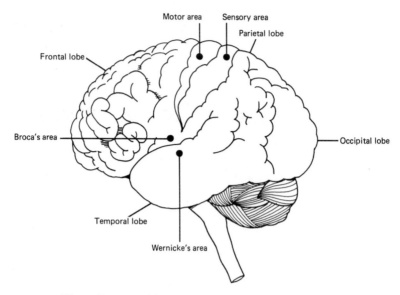

Figure 7.1 Lateral view of brain showing speech areas.

motor aspects of speech. This involves turning messages that are conceived in the brain into grammatically appropriate, smoothly coordinated speech patterns. The third major area controlling communication is the angular gyrus in the parietal lobe, which serves as an integration center for all incoming sensory systems; visual, auditory, and tactile information is interpreted and related to language.

Damage to any or all of these areas or their connecting fibers can result in a condition called *aphasia*. Aphasia is an impairment of language which can include understanding or expression of words and ideas, or difficulty in reading, writing, or calculating. Any of these dysfunctions can occur alone or in combinations. Aphasia is also related to cerebral dominance. In 93 to 97% of people, speech control is located in the dominant left cerebral hemisphere. Therefore, many patients who have a stroke in the left hemisphere with right-sided hemiplegia will also have aphasia. Most patients with a stroke in the right hemisphere will have left-sided hemiplegia and no language problems. The main exception to this rule seems to be left-handed people. A significant number of left-handed people have their speech functions in the right hemisphere, which is also their dominant motor hemisphere.

Expressive Aphasia

Expressive aphasia, *Broca's aphasia*, and *motor aphasia* are all terms used to describe the same phenomenon that occurs as a result of damage to Broca's area. The person with this language disorder understands incoming messages and knows what response to make, but has difficulty in expressing the reply. There is difficulty initiating speech, and when it finally comes, the thought is expressed in words or phrases, rarely complete sentences. The person with expressive aphasia tends to use nouns and verbs in their simplest form with no linking words. Thus, the speech sounds like "Me hurt" or "Wife come." Questions may be correctly answered with a yes or no. In its most severe form, expressive aphasia results in the inability to produce anything more than just sounds.

Three other circumstances are commonly present in patients with expressive aphasia. The first is difficulty with writing. The same problems are present in writing as in speech, ruling out written messages as an alternative means of communication. Second is the repetition of certain words or sounds, called *perseveration*. The few words the patient does have are repeated uncontrollably such as "now, now, now, now . . . ," a very frustrating situation for the patient. Third, some phrases or verses that we have overlearned in our lifetimes seem to be spoken spontaneously and without thought even by the aphasic patient. For example, counting to ten, naming the days of the week, saying "all right" or "you know" can often be done with no difficulty because they are so well learned that they have become automatic.

Receptive Aphasia

Receptive aphasia, Wernicke's aphasia, and *sensory aphasia* are all terms used to describe difficulties in comprehension. This person speaks very easily and words are formed without difficulty, but the speech has no meaning because there is no understanding of language. Wernicke's area in the brain has been damaged, that vital area which controls our ability to interpret language, both spoken and written. The patient with receptive aphasia may sound like a double-talk artist who forms words and sentences fluently and who sounds normal for a few seconds, before the listener realizes that the words are mostly an unrelated jumble. As with expressive aphasia, receptive aphasia occurs in varying degrees, from no comprehension or comprehensible language to less severe forms, where the worst problem may be difficulty in naming objects correctly.

Global Aphasia

With severe brain damage, both Broca's and Wernicke's areas and perhaps also the angular gyrus may be affected, with a combination of expressive and receptive aphasia resulting. The term for such a combination is *global aphasia*. It is seen most commonly in elderly people, and carries the poorest prognosis and the biggest problems, since all avenues of communication are cut off.

Table 7.1 summarizes the manifestations of the principal types of aphasia.

Dysarthria

Dysarthria is a speech difficulty related to aphasia, but is primarily an inability to speak because of impairment of the muscles of speech or their innervation. Paralysis or weakness of the lips, tongue, or pharynx results in slurred or garbled speech. Dysarthria is sometimes mistaken for expressive aphasia.

Apraxia

Apraxia is a broad term referring to the inability to perform a voluntary movement even though there is no weakness or paralysis. A particular movement that could not be carried out purposefully may be performed automatically at another time. For example, a patient may be unable to touch his or her nose on command, but when the nose itches, scratching occurs automatically. Lesions that cause apraxia may be found in various areas in either cerebral hemisphere.

Facial apraxia involves not only the inability to form words, but also difficulty drinking through a straw or chewing food on command. Although any of these actions may be performed spontaneously, the person cannot perform them when asked. Limb apraxia is also common;

TABLE 7.1 Manifestations of Aphasia

Type	Possible Symptoms
Expressive aphasia (Broca's aphasia; motor aphasia)	Difficulty expressing thoughts Understands incoming language Uses just nouns and verbs or single words Just produces sounds Perseveration of words Difficulty with writing
Receptive aphasia (Wernicke's aphasia; sensory aphasia)	Speaks fluently without making sense Makes up new words, uses words incorrectly Does not understand incoming language Difficulty naming objects Writing also lacks meaning
Global aphasia	No means of verbal communication No comprehension of language May express a few words with no meaning
Combined aphasias	Various combinations of expressive and receptive aphasia with possible alexia and agraphia

this person cannot perform limb movements on command. When making a diagnosis, the speech pathologist must differentiate between receptive aphasia and apraxia.

Alexia and Agraphia

Alexia, inability to read, and *agraphia*, inability to write, can occur singly or together and can occur in pure form or mixed with other aphasias. Alexia and agraphia result from damage to the visual cortex and the angular gyrus.

Combined Language Difficulties

The greatest problems encountered in diagnosing and treating language problems arise when the patient has combined symptoms. Patient A may have pure expressive aphasia, while Patient B has primarily expressive aphasia with some aspects of receptive aphasia and facial apraxia, and Patient C has dysarthria with mild receptive aphasia and agraphia. The speech pathologist is expert in diagnosing pure and combined problems; this is beyond the scope of nursing. However, the nurse must understand these diagnoses to provide appropriate care.

THE NURSE'S ROLE WITH APHASIC PATIENTS

Assessment

A speech pathologist will probably not see your aphasic patient until the medical condition has been stabilized. In the meantime, you must do simple assessments that will help you to recognize some of the patient's communication problems and abilities so that you can effectively communicate in some way with the patient.

Observe any attempts the patient makes to speak. Listen to the content of the speech; does it make sense, and is it grammatically correct? Are the words clear or slurred? If slurred, watch the face closely for muscular weakness or hemiplegia. Check for difficulty in sucking or chewing, which may also be signs of muscular weakness.

Evaluate the patient's ability to comprehend your speech. Are yes-and-no questions answered correctly? Does the patient carry out commands? If commands are not followed, check for the possibility of a hearing impairment. Ask the patient to name some items that you point to. (First make sure that there is no visual impairment.) If you suspect that the patient understands you but has expressive aphasia, you can name the item and have the patient point to it.

Assess the patient's reading and writing abilities in relation to pre-morbid abilities. Visual problems and hemiplegia may interfere with these assessments and must be taken into account. Another important assessment is of the person's ability to remember spoken language. Tell the patient three or four names of items and see if the names can be repeated back to you in the same order. If not, the patient may be unable to remember your verbal instructions, either.

Assessments should be done every day in the period of initial illness, because great changes in abilities may occur in short periods of time. These assessments must also be documented on the chart so that the patient is not needlessly bothered by questions from every nurse who comes in.

Approach to the Patient

Our minds often conceive of people with language problems as being childlike, since young children have limited language function. We must be careful, therefore, not to yield to the temptation to talk to the aphasic adult as if talking to a child. This practice is belittling for the patient and can retard progress. For the same reason, the patient should not be made more dependent on the nurse than necessary. If we perceive the patient as childlike, nursing care will be geared toward this age level and may involve doing everything for the patient, regardless of his or her abilities.

The decrease in communication abilities will make the patient feel isolated from the rest of the world. So it is important to talk to the patient even if you get no response. Explain everything that you are doing and explain what is happening as far as the patient's condition is concerned. Tell the patient that the language problem is part of the disease or trauma sustained and that you will do everything you can to help make communicating easier. Adhering to a routine daily schedule of care will help the patient with receptive aphasia make more sense of the world and provide a feeling of security.

Be careful of what you say in the presence of a patient with receptive aphasia. Do not assume that the patient understands nothing, because you cannot know for sure. Rather than talking *about* the patient while you are in the room, talk *to* the patient and include him or her in the conversation. Another tendency that people have when dealing with aphasic patients is to shout at them, unconsciously trying to make them understand better by raising the voice. Not only does shouting not help, but it is irritating and embarrassing for the patient.

Patients with receptive aphasia may mask their lack of understanding by smiling or nodding and looking attentive while you are speaking. Do not assume that the patient comprehends just because you get a smile in response. The patient may be responding to your tone of voice or your gestures rather than to your words. If you assume that your message has been received when in fact it has not, you will only compound the patient's problems. Check to see if the patient understands by giving a command and seeing if it is carried out. It is important for the nurse to be honest and admit it when it is impossible to understand what the patient is trying to say. Do not pretend that you understand or just smile or say yes. Instead, encourage the patient to find an alternative way to convey the message.

A great deal of patience is needed in working with aphasic patients. The nurse needs to give the patient time to understand what is going on and to take time to listen to the sometimes tortured speech. Studies have shown that patients are well aware of nurses' impatience and desire to get away and do something else. Body language can get a message across very quickly, and if the nurse keeps looking at the clock while the patient tries to speak, the message will be clear.

The most important aspect of your approach to this patient is your understanding. Try to understand the patient's plight and emotional responses to it. Be empathetic when the person is depressed or frustrated or tearful. Remember, too, that these patients are often confronted with multiple problems. To experience pain and fearful procedures is bad enough, but when you cannot talk about it, the situation becomes overwhelming.

Setting Up a System of Communication

Aphasia is usually at its worst in the first few days after a stroke or injury. During this initial period, it may be difficult to communicate in any way with the patient. The simplest means of communication is through gestures and pantomime. Pointing at items and acting out certain requests may be helpful in getting messages through to severely aphasic patients, and they in turn may be able to use pointing and gestures to make their needs known.

The next method to try is picture cards portraying hospital items or situations, such as a bedpan, a meal tray, or a family visiting. The patient with severe expressive aphasia may be able to point to or select the appropriate card to communicate a need or a question. If this technique works, write a nursing order in the card file (Kardex) to "Use picture cards for patient to point to." If you have determined that the individual can answer yes-and-no questions accurately, use this channel of communication, asking all questions so they can be answered yes or no. Once greater language function returns, however, you should encourage more speech than just one-word answers.

As more understanding develops and more speech returns, the

patient may be able to express basic needs by saying a few nouns and verbs. At this point, picture cards and gestures should be used only when absolutely necessary. By taking time and listening carefully, you may be able to understand the patient's speech, especially as you get used to it. It also helps the patient to understand you better if you talk at eye level rather than standing above the patient. Keep your sentences and questions short and to the point at this stage. Extra words may only confuse the patient.

When you are attempting to converse with the patient, limit other stimuli in the environment. The person will stand a better chance of focusing on your message if there are no other distractions around, such as television, people walking by, or voices speaking over an inter-com.

Encouraging Speech

When the period of acute illness is over and the patient's condition is stable, the nurse should continue using whatever system of communi-cation has already been established, while encouraging the patient to use more words and to identify more objects in the environment.

Time should be set aside during the day for helping the patient with language rehabilitation, but short sessions should be used so that the patient does not become fatigued. You do not have to limit these sessions to communication. You can encourage speech while giving the patient a bath or while doing range-of-motion exercises. Just make sure that you are not introducing too many stimuli at the same time, since overstimulation will interfere with the person's concentration.

One way of encouraging speech is to talk about an activity that the patient is performing or that you yourself are doing. Describe the range-of-motion exercises that you are doing with the patient. The patient will hear your words and learn to associate them with the actions that can be seen or felt. Encourage the patient to arrange his or her own lunch tray and describe the foods and actions that you see. Linking words to actions that can be seen or felt can help the person to regain language skills through other sensory avenues, rather than relying only on audi-tory perception, which may be impaired.

You should also stimulate the patient's use of words. This can be done by asking the names of items that you point to. Sometimes you may have to name the item first, and have the patient repeat after you. If the patient makes a mistake, do not correct it, but just follow up by using the word correctly yourself. If the individual cannot get the word out, try starting the first syllable yourself and encourage the patient to complete the word. You can then have the patient try to repeat the en-tire word. Another alternative to use if a patient is having difficulty finding the right word is to offer choices of a few words. Have the patient select the correct word, just as in a multiple-choice question.

Initially, patients with expressive aphasia will talk with only nouns and verbs. You can encourage speech by filling out the patient's sentence with some of the connecting and modifying words. For example, if the patient says, "Me go walk," you can fill out the sentence and say "You want to go for a walk in the hall?" Just as a child learns to speak by listening to others talking, so can the aphasic person relearn speech by hearing other people.

Speech pathologists have done some research in the use of music therapy for aphasics. Some patients, it seems, may be able to sing the words they want to say, better than they can speak them. This may be an avenue that nurses can use in the future to help encourage speech.

It is important that you give the patient time to get thoughts together and to get the words out. If you ask a question, give ample time for the person to express an answer. Learn to be comfortable with some silence and some hard work on the part of the patient. Do not belabor an answer that will not come, however, because a lot of frustration can retard progress. Praise any efforts that the patient makes and any success that is achieved.

Since the patient will be listening to and imitating your speech, you should be careful to provide a good example. Your sentences should be short, but with good grammatical structure. Pronounce words clearly and distinctly, speaking more slowly than usual, but not exaggerating your words.

Evaluation

After you have instituted some of the above-mentioned approaches to communication, evaluate the system you have set up. Can the patient communicate his or her needs? Has there been any improvement in communication? Has the patient's frustration decreased? Are all staff members following the same plan? Have your goals been met to any degree?

The evaluation process will reveal any weaknesses in your plans and interventions and may indicate the need for revisions in your care. Maybe you will have to continue using picture cards longer than you had planned, or maybe you will realize that you have to do more to encourage the patient to speak. Revise your nursing orders and try again.

Helping the Patient's Family

Imagine how upset your patient's family must be when the full impact of aphasia hits them. They can no longer communicate normally with their loved one and may fear that the situation will never change.

They need explanations about what has happened and what will be done to help the patient.

You must include the family when establishing a plan for communicating with the patient. Since they are more familiar with the patient's premorbid personality, habits, and interests, they can contribute valuable information about how to help this patient. If you are attempting to encourage speech, for example, centering the conversation around hobbies and interests may motivate the patient to want to contribute to the conversation.

Teaching the family about language rehabilitation measures will serve two purposes. First, it will help them to help the patient in improving speech. Second, it will help the family to feel that they are making a valuable contribution to their loved one's recovery. The more the family knows about the patient's aphasia and approaches to communication, the more likely they are to try to talk *to* the patient rather than *about* the patient while they are visiting. An uninformed family often considers the situation hopeless and excludes the patient from any conversation.

PROGNOSIS FOR APHASIC PATIENTS

Recovery from aphasia depends on several factors, including the extent of cerebral pathology, the patient's motivation to get well, premorbid use of language, and assistance or support from people around the patient. A tremendous amount of improvement may be seen in the first few weeks after the onset of aphasia; in fact, if there is no improvement in those first few weeks, the prognosis for recovery is poor. It is possible for aphasia to clear up completely in a week or two, but if significant language disturbance persists without improvement for more than a few weeks, the patient will probably always have residual language deficits.

For a period of up to 6 months, the aphasic patient may continue to improve at a rapid pace; after that, recovery may be slower, but can continue for over 2 years. Speech therapy is valuable during this time because detailed assessments are made that pinpoint the patient's deficits, and extensive plans are established to help the patient communicate. The speech pathologist is an expert who can best help the patient to reestablish good language habits and who can prescribe specific exercises and programs that are tailored for the individual patient.

The condition with the poorest prognosis is global aphasia. If no improvement is seen within a few days, there has probably been such widespread destruction of the cerebral language areas that recovery is not likely. Although it is possible that thinking abilities are retained, this person is left without any sufficient means of communication with the world.

Prognosis for the bilingual patient is difficult to predict. Deficits will occur for both languages, but one may be spared more than the other. The language in which the patient was more fluent will probably be better preserved, but sometimes the more recently learned and used language is spared even though the patient has used it for less time.

The patient's ability to recognize his or her own speech errors is considered a favorable sign for remission of aphasia. Recognizing and correcting errors requires clear thought processes and motivation; the fact that the patient makes such an effort makes the prognosis much more optimistic. Do not be surprised, though, if the patient is aware of errors one day and not the next, or can speak a full sentence one hour and not the next. The course of aphasia is very variable, with many periods of improvement followed by worsening of symptoms, in an unpredictable pattern. This vacillation is peculiar to the disease process and can be expected to some degree in all aphasics. Therefore, you should not measure improvement on an hourly or daily basis, but must look for long-term trends.

SPEECH ALTERATIONS IN NEUROMUSCULAR DISORDERS

Changes in Respiratory Activity

Reduced chest excursion, decreased vital capacity, weakness of the diaphragm, and improper closing of the glottis are all dysfunctions that are found in neuromuscular disorders and which can affect speech. People with cerebral palsy, Parkinson's disease, amyotrophic lateral sclerosis, and myasthenia gravis can be affected by one or all of these respiratory problems. As a result, speech can be intermittent, changed in pitch, or variable in volume. Changes in volume of speech may make it difficult to understand the patient. Alternating loudness and softness interferes with the listener's ability to follow the speech. The most distressing voice change is persistent low volume, which makes the speech sound mumbled and garbled.

Changes in Intonation and Rate of Speech

Victims of Parkinson's disease are particularly prone to monotony and rapid rate of speech. They do not emphasize the proper syllables or words in a sentence; this lack of inflection makes the speech very regular, flat, and uninteresting to listen to. Although some people with

Parkinson's have a very slow rate of speech, most have an increased rate, with the rate becoming increasingly faster near the end of a sentence or thought. The combination of monotony and speed makes the speech seem a run of unintelligible words.

Scanning Speech

Scanning speech is a phenomenon seen primarily in multiple sclerosis. It consists of prolonged intervals between syllables and between words, as well as even emphasis on all syllables and words. The result sounds very halting and monotonous. Scanning speech is sometimes referred to as *ataxic dysarthria.*

Nursing Interventions

The patient with speech problems due to neuromuscular disturbances may not benefit from therapy to any great extent, since the effort it would take the patient to correct the problems would require too much energy on a sustained basis. There are, however, some limited approaches that can be used.

Instruct the patient in some exercises that will help maintain function of the facial muscles. Such movements as pursing the lips, smiling, sticking out the tongue, and whistling will help the patient to keep control of the muscles of speech. If the patient reads aloud at intervals throughout the day, the muscles will also be exercised and the patient may be able to correct errors and practice breath control.

Rapid speech rate and mumbling seen in Parkinson's disease may improve somewhat if you encourage the patient to speak slowly and exaggerate the lip movements. If low volume is the major problem, the patient may benefit from an electronic amplifier of the type used by laryngectomees. If this approach is not feasible, you can at least get as close to the patient as possible in order to catch the words.

EMOTIONAL IMPLICATIONS OF ALTERED COMMUNICATION

A variety of emotional responses may be encountered in patients who have sustained cerebral injury that affects communication. After the period of acute injury, patients who improve physically but are left with language deficits may go through a period of emotional euphoria. At this stage the patient realizes how close the brush with death was and is elated to have come through so well. The realities of the language difficulty are denied or not yet fully appreciated.

If there is little appreciable improvement in speech over the next few weeks, the patient tends to become depressed and easily frustrated. The same reaction is seen in patients with degenerative neurological problems, such as multiple sclerosis. The knowledge that the speech difficulties, in this case, are unlikely to go away and will probably become worse leads to understandable depression.

Individuals with receptive aphasia may exhibit inappropriate emotional responses because their understanding of the situation is limited. They are often in a happier state than their situation would warrant, as long as their basic needs are being met and they are comfortable. But they may have paranoid reactions when they see their listeners grinning or looking embarrassed in response to the double-talk or nonsense words that they are saying. They cannot understand why people around them seem to be making fun of them.

Severe impairment of understanding can lead to disturbing changes in behavior. The patient who cannot make sense of the environment and cannot communicate with others in that environment may become very fearful or very angry. This results in restlessness or combative behavior. The patient does not allow procedures to be done and does not trust the nurses, doctors, or technicians.

In most cases of communication impairment, patients respond emotionally in accordance with their premorbid personalities. So if an individual has always been an optimist and an indomitable spirit, he or she will react more positively and with greater motivation than an individual who tended to be a pessimist and a victim of despair.

What can the nurse do to help patients with these emotional changes due to impaired communication? Besides the attempts to set up an improved system of communication, there are several interventions the nurse can use.

The first rule must be to accept the patient's behavior, whatever it is. If you realize that the patient does not wish to respond in such a way, but is being controlled somewhat by the pathology and the physical limitations of the illness, it becomes easier to deal with the situation. Telling the patient that you understand how upsetting and frustrating it must be to be unable to communicate may help to reduce some of the patient's anxiety.

Touching is a means of communication that the patient may find very reassuring. Touching the person's hand or shoulder can be a way of saying that you care and wish to help. If used in conjunction with a warm tone of voice and a calm manner, touch can help to alleviate emotional problems. If touch seems to be effective in reassuring your patient, record it as a nursing order in your care plan.

It is especially important to avoid embarrassing a patient who speaks in a way that can seem amusing. Do not repeat nonsense phrases or jargon that the patient uses, or mimic the abnormal inflections that you hear. Monitor all your responses to make sure that the paranoid patient cannot construe them as amusement or unkindness. Be very careful when you talk to coworkers about the patient to make sure that you cannot be overheard.

Part of the nurse's role is to act as liaison person with other departments of the health care facility to smooth the way for the patient. If you know that the patient must go to x-ray or physical therapy, let that department know in advance about the patient's language problems and how they can communicate with the patient. If necessary, you may have to accompany the patient to avoid subjecting the patient to embarrassing and frustrating situations.

Communication disorders are often difficult to manage from a nursing perspective and require all the nurse's compassion and creativity to keep the patient in touch with society.

EXAMPLES OF NURSING DIAGNOSES RELATED TO ALTERED COMMUNICATION

Impaired verbal communication related to stroke; seems to understand but responds only with yes and no.

Receptive aphasia related to stroke; speaks fluent jargon but does not understand language.

Total impairment of verbal communication related to brain damage; communicates through gestures.

Impaired verbal communication related to weak facial muscles and slurred speech.

Impaired verbal communication related to persistently low volume of voice.

Anxiety related to inability to understand language.

Inability to read or write due to stroke.

Altered self-concept related to childlike use of language.

REFERENCES

Boone, Daniel R., *An Adult Has Aphasia*. Danville, Ill.: The Interstate Printers and Publishers, Inc., 1965.

Dreher, Barbara, "Overcoming Speech and Language Disorders," *Geriatric Nursing*, 2, no. 5 (September–October 1981), p. 345.

Fowler, Roy S., and Wilbert E. Fordyce, "Adapting Care for the Brain-

Damaged Patient," *American Journal of Nursing*, 72, no. 10 (October 1972), p. 1832.

Fox, Madeline, "Patients with Receptive Aphasia: They Really Don't Understand," *American Journal of Nursing*, 76, no. 10 (October 1976), p. 1596.

Gardner, Howard, *The Shattered Mind—The Person after Brain Damage*. New York: Alfred A. Knopf, Inc., 1975.

Norman, Susan, and Robin Baratz, "Understanding Aphasia," *American Journal of Nursing*, 79, no. 12 (December 1979), p. 2135.

O'Brien, Mary T., and Phyllis J. Pallett, *Total Care of the Stroke Patient*. Boston: Little, Brown and Company, 1978.

Piotrowski, Marcia, "Aphasia: Providing Better Nursing Care," *Nursing Clinics of North America*, 13, no. 3 (September 1978), p. 543.

Sarno, Martha Taylor, ed., *Aphasia: Selected Readings*. New York: Appleton-Century-Crofts, 1972.

8

Sensory and Perceptual Alterations

Neurologic patients with alterations of sensation or perception often receive little help with these problems. There are several reasons for this. The patient may have so many other problems of higher priority that sensory and perceptual dysfunctions are relegated to the end of the list. Also, such problems are sometimes difficult to detect and the health care team may not be aware that they exist. Third, these are fairly new areas of study and investigation, and not a lot of medical or nursing interventions are available to assist the patient, making in-depth assessment sometimes seem futile.

With the knowledge that we do have, however, we can be of some assistance to the patient with sensory and perceptual alterations. We can use our assessment techniques to identify the problem clearly and then plan ways of helping the patient adjust to the situation and ways of preventing injury and frustration that can result from these dysfunctions.

This chapter includes a discussion of pathological processes resulting in problems of sensation and problems of perception. It will explore nursing interventions that are known to be of some help in coping with sensory and perceptual problems.

ALTERATIONS IN SENSATION

Changes in sensation that may be experienced by the neurologic patient include paresthesia, loss of sensation, and pain.

Paresthesia

Paresthesias, abnormal sensations such as tingling, crawling, or burn-ing feelings, frequently accompany demyelinating diseases such as mul-tiple sclerosis. The sensations are usually transient in such cases, but can be very distressing while they last. Paresthesias are also seen as a result of incomplete peripheral nerve damage due to injury or tumors. If a pe-ripheral nerve were completely severed, there would be a total loss of sensation, but partial interruption can cause a decrease in sensation, de-velopment of abnormal sensation, or an actual increase in sensation or increased sensitivity to stimuli. Paresthesias resulting from trauma may be temporary or permanent.

Nursing interventions. We can do very little to help the patient who suffers with burning or tingling of a body part. Interventions that work with some patients may be totally ineffective for others, and only trial and error may reveal some approaches that help.

You can try massaging the skin lightly with lotion, but usually this helps only while you are actually doing it; the effect does not last. In some cases, the patient cannot tolerate anything touching the part, and the best you can do is to place bed linen and clothing so that the area is completely uncovered.

Distracting the patient's attention away from the paresthesia may be the only successful intervention. Involve the person in conversation or some activity that will draw attention away from the problem. Night-time is often the worst for the patient because there is no distraction for the mind, so the paresthesia becomes the intolerable focus of attention. In this case you may have to administer an analgesic or sedative to en-able the patient to rest.

Loss of Sensation

Anesthesia, or absence of sensation, is at times a desirable condi-tion, but it may also be an unwanted companion to several neurologic dysfunctions, and it creates its own problems.

Pathways of sensation. Superficial sensations such as touch, pressure, vibration, position sense, temperature, and pain are all conducted by neurons from the periphery of the body to the spinal nerve roots. Each nerve root supplies one specific area of the body, called a *dermatome* (see Figure 8.1). The sensations are then divided up to be carried to the brain by several different nerve tracts.

An important nerve tract that carries fibers for fine touch, position sense (proprioception), and vibration is the *dorsal column*. It is known

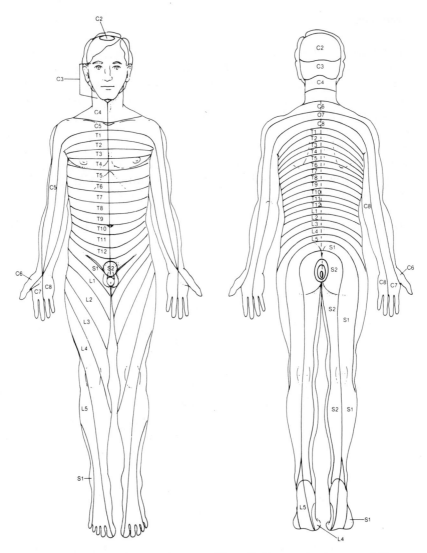

Figure 8.1 Dermatomes. (From William F. Evans, *Anatomy and Physiology*, 2nd ed., ©1976, p. 178. Reprinted by permission of Prentice-Hall, Inc., Englewood Cliffs, N.J.)

to cross over from one side of the spinal cord to the other in the medulla. The *lateral spinothalamic tract* conducts sensations of pain and temperature and the *ventral spinothalamic tract* carries fibers for crude touch and pressure. The spinothalamic tracts cross over from one side of the cord to the other immediately upon entering the cord. These sensory tracts all terminate in the thalamus. Projection fibers then connect the thalamus to the primary sensory cortex in the parietal lobe.

Pathology.   The type and extent of sensory loss that is caused by various pathological processes relates to the location of the lesion in the brain, spinal cord, or periphery of the body. A stroke can cause varied sensory losses depending on the location of the cerebral infarct. If parts of the primary sensory cortex are affected, any combination of effects is possible, to any degree on one side of the body. If part of the thalamus is damaged, there may be complete contralateral anesthesia.

Complete spinal cord transection results in complete anesthesia below the level of the lesion. Incomplete spinal cord lesions or spinal cord tumors may affect one or more tracts with effects such as loss of pain and temperature on one side of the body below the lesion, loss of touch and pressure sensation on one side, or loss of pain and temperature on one side and loss of touch and pressure on the other side.

Surgical procedures performed to relieve intractable pain attempt to interrupt the sensory pathways at some point. It may be at a peripheral nerve site or in the spinal cord, where a sensory tract may be destroyed. Again, depending on the location of the lesion that is made, just pain and temperature sensations may be interrupted, or all sensation may be blocked.

If you are familiar with the sensory pathways, you will begin to understand the varying sensory losses your patient may have.

Nursing implications.   Patients who have lost sensation in large areas of their bodies may feel very deprived of the feeling of being touched by other people. This is especially true for quadriplegic patients, who may have no sensory function below the shoulders. Because touching is a sign of caring, you should make an effort to touch these patients occasionally to provide sensory input from intact areas and to offer comfort.

Loss of the sensations of touch and pressure can have physical as well as emotional consequences. Normally, we experience discomfort if we do not change position and if pressure on one area of the skin is prolonged. Deprived of this sensation, we are not aware of prolonged pressure and the damage it may be causing. Therefore, protection of the skin must be carried out by routine position changes and by inspecting the skin carefully once or twice a day. People who have lost sensation over the back and buttocks should be taught to check the skin over those areas by using mirrors.

When the senses of touch, pain, and proprioception are lost, the patient becomes extra injury prone. Trauma of various types, such as cuts, bruises, and excoriations, may be sustained but not felt. You must protect the patient as well as teach self-protection. Make sure that hands and elbows are inside a wheelchair when going through a doorway. Check the position of the legs and feet before having the patient stand. Inspect all the fingers after the person uses a knife or scissors. The individual must be taught always to check the position of insensitive extremities before moving, and periodically to inspect the areas without sensation for any damage.

Loss of temperature sensation can lead to damage from burns or frostbite. Again, patient teaching is essential. Scalding by hot water can happen very easily if the skin is insensitive. The person should learn to test the water on normal skin, or use a bath thermometer. Ironing must be done with caution if there is loss of temperature sensation in the hands or arms. When working around a stove, pot holders or oven mits should always be used. Heating pads are a common source of burns and should only be used on a low setting and with proper skin protection. In cold weather, enough layers of warm clothing must be worn to protect the skin from frostbite.

Pain

The experience of pain is, in a sense, a normal phenomenon, in that we have nerves and nerve tracts in our bodies specifically placed for the purpose of carrying pain messages. Yet, when we experience pain it is by no means a normal thing, but rather a warning of something that is wrong, and a situation from which we want to escape.

Unfortunately, pain is a common occurrence for many neurologic patients. Those having diagnostic tests or undergoing surgery suffer at least short-term pain. Patients with head injuries or brain tumors experience headaches. The pain of muscle spasms can be excruciating and may persist for a long time. Pain from contractures can be seen in many patients with severe neurologic impairment. Injury or disease of the peripheral nerves can lead to unbearable chronic pain.

Pain is classified as acute or chronic depending upon the length of time it has existed. Pain that lasts less than 6 months is usually defined as *acute pain*, anything lasting longer than that is *chronic pain*. Whereas the cause of acute pain is often known, chronic pain may be of unknown etiology.

A further way of categorizing pain is according to whether its origins are in the peripheral nerves or in the central nervous system. *Peripheral pain* includes such entities as low back pain, trigeminal neuralgia, and *causalgia*, pain occurring as a result of injury to a peripheral nerve. *Central pain* consists of problems such as pain from spinal cord injury, multiple sclerosis (rare), or brain tumor.

Nursing management. The nurse's attitude toward a patient's pain influences assessment and intervention modalities. Sometimes it is very obvious that a patient is in great pain, for example, in a case of trigeminal neuralgia. When there are obvious physiologic signs of pain and the patient cannot hide the distress it causes, the nurse is likely to feel compassion and do anything possible to try to relieve the pain. But when there are no physiologic signals and the patient does not exhibit any great distress, as in many cases of chronic pain, the nurse is apt not to believe in the patient's pain or its severity and offer little nursing support.

Before you can help any patient in pain you must believe that pain is a subjective sensation and that you have to take the patient's word for its presence and severity. Many patients with chronic pain have adapted to it to the point where they do not show distress and are able to function; this does not mean the pain is not there.

Because pain is subjective, your assessment of it will depend to the greatest extent on what the patient tells you. You may look for some objective signs, such as muscle tension, sweating, tachycardia, and clenched hands, but the descriptive information must come from the patient. Ask about the exact location of the pain and possible radiation to other areas. Get the patient to describe the pain's quality—whether sharp, dull, throbbing, stabbing, crushing, etc. Find out if certain movements or circumstances bring on the pain or increase its severity. It is also important to assess the effect of the pain on the patient. Is it causing fear or anxiety, depression or despair? Is the patient using any coping mechanisms or support systems to help bear the pain? Are there any means by which the patient is able to relieve the pain? Sometimes we overlook the home remedies that patients use successfully, especially for chronic pain.

Once you have done your assessment, you can plan which interventions you are going to use. There are many independent nursing measures that you can employ to alleviate pain, as well as some measures that are carried out in conjunction with the physician. Recent research has shown us that some of the simple nursing measures, such as changing position, giving a back rub, and helping the patient to relax, which have been downplayed in recent years, may actually have scientific value.

Scientists have discovered a group of polypeptides with opiatelike characteristics, called *endorphins*, which are normally present in the nervous system and seem to inhibit or modify pain messages that are on their way to the brain. Although some of the findings are still tentative, it seems that endorphin release can be stimulated by many of the measures we use to alleviate pain.

Giving a back rub or massaging a painful area may not just be psychologically soothing but may stimulate endorphin release, which will help to reduce the patient's pain. If you explain this action to your patient, you may get even better results, because the patient will have greater faith in that back rub than ever before.

Chronic pain, anxiety, and depression all seem to suppress or deplete the endorphins. We know that all pain is accompanied by some anxiety. Therefore, if we can reduce the patient's anxiety, we may permit the endorphins to take over some of their pain-relieving work again. There are several ways in which we can help to reduce the anxiety of a patient in pain.

Explanations and information given to a patient can take away some of the fear of the unknown and thus reduce anxiety. Explanations about the cause of the pain and assurance that pain relief is possible will also eliminate some fear.

Use of breath control can be very effective in helping a patient to relax. Tell the patient to breathe to the slow count of 1-2-3 on inspiration and 1-2-3-4 on expiration. Help the patient to concentrate on breathing to a steady comfortable pattern, with an occasional sigh. Control of breathing and concentration on it reduces anxiety, relaxes muscles, and helps the patient to gain some control. If you have found a pattern that works well with your patient, explain it in a nursing order on your care plan.

Other relaxation techniques are also valuable, but may take more of your time. They can be used to help the patient with chronic pain, even at home. Most of these techniques involve breath control, concentration on relaxing specific muscle groups one at a time, and using the imagination to picture a favorite place or restful scene. You can investigate the work of Margo McCaffery and other experts in pain relief for details on relaxation techniques.

Distraction techniques are invaluable in helping anyone with pain. If you can draw the patient's thoughts away from the pain and provide other sensory input, the perception of the pain is at least temporarily modified. If you have extra time, spend it with the patient. Conversation is one of the best distractions. Enlist the help of other patients and family members to distract the patient's thoughts. Television and radio may be helpful, as well as books or crafts. Humor and laughter are great distractions and do much to relieve pain.

Changing a patient's position seems like an obvious thing to do when a patient experiences pain, but it is often not done because the patient does not want to move, and nurses do not think of movement as a way of relieving pain. Repositioning reduces muscle tension and fatigue and generally helps the patient to relax.

Several skin stimulation techniques are available for pain relief. The oldest modality is probably the application of heat. People have long been aware that heat application reduces many types of pain. Sometimes this is due to the increase in blood flow through the area; perhaps it is also related to the theory that any stimulation of peripheral nerves modifies the perception of pain that is already there; and it may be effective because it stimulates endorphin release.

Another popular theory that explains why heat and other methods of skin stimulation help relieve pain is the *gate control theory*. This theory proposes that there are two types of nerve fibers, large- and small-diameter fibers. Large-diameter fibers prevent pain; small-diameter fibers facilitate pain. If the large fibers are stimulated, they can "close the gate" in the spinal cord and prevent impulses from the small fibers from getting through to the brain. Since the skin contains many large-diameter nerve fibers, it lends itself to stimulation techniques that will close the gate on the pain.

Other skin stimulation methods that help alleviate pain include the application of cold packs, pressure over or near the affected area, or external analgesics which are rubbed into the painful area. A newer treatment is electrical stimulation, or the use of battery-operated pain suppressors (see Figure 8.2). Of course, this intervention requires a doctor's order, but nurses are becoming more involved in helping patients to learn to operate the equipment successfully. In electrical stimulation, mild electric current is given to the skin by means of electrodes. The amount of current needed to control pain can be adjusted by the patient. When pain is felt, the current is turned on and the patient may experience a vibration or tingling sensation, but no pain. The pain relief may last for hours after a few minutes of current.

The electrodes are usually placed near or right over the painful part and a conductive gel or warm water is applied under the electrodes. Tape

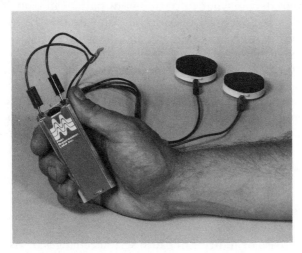

Figure 8.2 Battery-operated pain suppressor. (Reprinted by permission; ©J. A. Preston Corp., 1981.)

or a belt can be used to hold the electrodes in place. If the apparatus is being used continuously, the electrodes should be removed once a day and the skin cleansed. If possible, the electrodes should be replaced over a different skin area.

Too often nurses neglect all these interventions for pain and rely just on analgesics. Not that analgesics are not good and valuable, but we should not ignore all the other interventions that can be used *together with* analgesics. Both nonnarcotic and narcotic analgesics are widely used and are very effective, especially if you give the medication with a positive attitude that it *will* help to reduce the pain.

Analgesics are usually ordered on a p.r.n. basis, typically every 4 hours p.r.n. Some nurses have the idea that if a 4-hour interval is good, 6 hours would be better, and they try to withhold the drug as long as possible, perhaps fearing that the patient will become dependent on it. There is usually little danger of addiction, except in some cases of chronic pain, and it may do harm to withhold the drug beyond the 4 hours. Analgesics are most effective if given before the pain and anxiety have become severe.

Some of the commonly used analgesics also have commonly occurring side effects of which you must be aware. Watch for signs of dizziness, respiratory depression, nausea, vomiting, and constipation after giving narcotics. Check for tinnitus, bruising, and melena if giving a lot of aspirin. There are many other effects accompanying individual drugs that you should check in the drug literature.

With all these interventions from which to choose, it may be difficult for you to decide what to try for your patient in pain. Your choice may be guided by the location of the pain, its severity, the patient's personality and attitude toward pain, and by your consultation with the physician. Sometimes trial-and-error tactics are necessary.

Record your plan and any modifications of it on the care plan. Modifications are made after you have tried some interventions and evaluated the results. If the intervention has not relieved the pain at all, nor the anxiety, nor helped the patient to relax, it is time to modify the intervention or switch to another approach. If nursing interventions are unsuccessful in relieving or abating the pain, consult with the physician about further medical intervention.

VISUAL ALTERATIONS

Neurologic disease or injury can cause serious changes in vision, notably *diplopia* and *homonymous hemianopsia*. Diplopia is seen most often in multiple sclerosis, myasthenia gravis, or cranial nerve diseases. It usually results from damage to the oculomotor nerve, although the trochlear and abducens may also be implicated. Because of muscle weakness, the eyes fail to coordinate in their movements, and thus do not focus on the same point at the same time, leaving the patient with diplopia (double vision). In the case of multiple sclerosis, the diplopia often goes into remission.

Homonymous hemianopsia is a visual field disorder associated with stroke, brain tumors, or cerebral trauma. It is caused by damage to the optic nerve posterior to the optic chiasm. Figure 8.3 demonstrates that a lesion, for example, on the right side of the brain posterior to the optic chiasm results in a visual field loss in the nasal half of the right eye and temporal half of the left eye. Therefore, a stroke patient with right cerebral damage and left hemiplegia may very well lose the left field of vision. The opposite will occur with left cerebral damage; the patient will have right homonymous hemianopsia with no vision out of the right side of either eye.

Homonymous hemianopsia goes undetected in many patients until after the acute stage of illness, because up until then, mental confusion or decreased awareness and communication difficulties may have interfered with the patient's ability to recognize and report the problem. In fact, unless a nurse or physician actually assesses the visual fields with

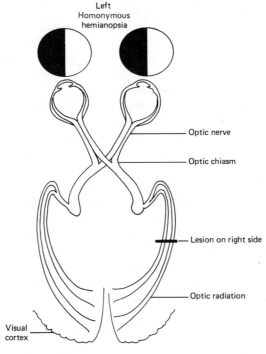

Figure 8.3 Visual pathways and visual fields with a lesion causing left homonymous hemianopsia.

the confrontation test or similar methods, the visual field cut may not be noticed until the patient begins to show signs such as ignoring activity on one side of the bed, or having to turn the head frequently to one side to see what is going on.

Nursing Interventions

Whether the visual alterations are temporary or permanent, there are a few things you can do to help the patient cope with the defects and see as much of the environment as possible.

Patients with diplopia are usually treated with an eye patch over one eye. This method very simply eliminates the double vision. However, the patch should not be used on just one eye because an unused eye can suffer loss of visual acuity. Rather, the patch should be changed from one eye to the other a few times a day. When nurses are responsible for switching the patch, a nursing order should appear on the care plan stating, "Change patch to alternate eye Q4H" and a schedule may even be listed.

Nursing approaches used for homonymous hemianopsia include careful arrangement of the patient's environment, visual field scanning to compensate for the loss, and visual exercises.

The patient's room should be arranged so that the patient's unaffected side faces the door, or the part of a room where activity is taking place. This arrangement allows for the greatest amount of sensory input and prevents the patient from feeling isolated. You should place all articles that the patient uses on the unaffected side so they can be seen. When you approach the patient to talk or provide care, approach from the unaffected side. Sometimes, during the later phases of rehabilitation, it may be appropriate to work from the patient's affected side to force the patient to be alert to the whole environment and to compensate for the visual field.

Visual field scanning is a device the patient can learn to use with some practice. Have the patient turn his or her head toward the blind side and scan the whole area to get the picture of what is going on. Scanning prevents problems such as walking into objects, ignoring people, and not seeing items on an overbed table. During mealtimes and bath time, scanning permits the patient to be more independent.

Exercises can be done with the patient to teach compensation for the visual loss. Reading exercises are very helpful. The patient can follow along the lines with a finger to make sure that no words near the margin are missed. A colored guide can be placed along the margin to remind the patient where the line begins or ends.

ALTERATIONS IN PERCEPTION

Some patients with brain damage from injury or stroke retain normal sensation, but when they receive sensory messages, they cannot interpret and integrate them to make a meaningful whole. This phenomenon is called *perceptual deficit*, and is seen most frequently in the presence of damage to the right cerebral hemisphere. It is the right hemisphere that is mostly responsible for perception, including the sense of spatial proportion, distance and rate perception, ability to recognize faces and familiar objects, perception of time, and ability to follow visual instructions. When perceptual deficits are added to other problems of brain-damaged patients, such as hemiplegia, hemianesthesia, and perhaps homonymous hemianopsia, you can understand why the patient has difficulty making sense of the environment.

Manifestations of Perceptual Alterations

One of the most common perceptual deficits is difficulty judging space, distance, and rate of movement (see Table 8.1). This kind of deficit makes the patient prone to accidents from bumping into objects, hitting doorways with a wheelchair, and knocking over dishes on a table. Lack of depth perception adds to the problem. The patient may reach for a safety handle to lean on, only to find that it is another 6 inches away. Lack of balance is also sometimes attributed to spatial distortions. Confusion over directions, such as left and right or up and down, occurs frequently. The patient cannot differentiate between these terms, and if told to hold the right arm up, may do nothing because of lack of understanding.

One-sided neglect is an interesting phenomenon that occurs in some patients with right hemisphere lesions, particularly those with left hemiplegia. The person simply denies the existence of the left side of the body and pays no attention to the left side of the environment. The problem may be so severe that a patient asked to draw a self-portrait will draw only one side of the body, and when eating from a tray, may eat only those foods on the right side of the tray. This deficit interferes not only with eating, but with all aspects of self-care. If may be accompanied by homonymous hemianopsia.

The inability to recognize familiar objects or faces is termed *agnosia*. Agnosias are classified according to the avenue of sensory input that is not being perceived. For example, if a patient cannot recognize a shoe or a loved one's face by sight, there is *visual agnosia*. If the patient, with eyes closed, cannot identify a toothbrush or spoon by the

TABLE 8.1 Assessment of Visual and Perceptual Deficits

Deficit	Means of Assessment
Homonymous hemianopsia	1. Observe for lack of attention paid to one side of room and for frequent head turning to that side.
	2. Perform confrontation test (see Chapter 2).
	3. Stand in front of patient, spread your arms wide, and move a finger of each hand into both temporal fields of vision. Watch patient's eyes for deviation. Ask how many fingers are seen.
Spatial deficits	1. Watch movement for clumsiness, bumping into furniture, knocking over small items.
	2. Ask patient to touch a small object that you hold out (may reveal disturbance in distance and depth perception).
	3. Have patient sit or stand in front of a long mirror. Ask patient to indicate when good posture and balance appear to exist (may reveal vertical distortions).
Left-right confusion	1. Ask patient to point to the left arm or right leg or left ear.
	2. Point to patient's left or right leg and ask which side it is.
One-sided neglect	1. Have patient try to read a full-width newspaper headline and see if words are left out on the affected side.
	2. Place about 10 small objects (comb, toothbrush, bobby pin) spread out on an overbed table. Seat patient behind the table and ask patient to name all the objects (patient may not name any objects on the neglected side).
Agnosia	1. Assess visual agnosia by asking patient to identify familiar people or objects only by sight.
	2. Assess tactile agnosia by having patient close the eyes, touch a familiar object, and try to identify it.
Apraxia	1. Ask patient to perform a routine self-care task such as brushing teeth or combing hair. If patient agrees to do so and is able to verbalize how to do so but does not proceed, apraxia may exist.

sense of touch alone, *tactile agnosia* exists. Tactile agnosia may occur only on the affected side of the body.

Apraxia is a deficit that occurs with either left or right hemisphere damage. The patient with apraxia is unable to carry out voluntary movements and activities even though he or she may be able to verbalize how to proceed, and even though all muscles are capable of functioning. If you ask the patient to put on a shirt, the patient agrees to do so, may be able to explain how to do it, but is unable to actually carry out the task. This is a very complex problem and is not yet fully understood.

Nursing Interventions for Perceptual Alterations

There are several ways in which you can help a patient with perceptual deficits in the realm of space, distance, and motion. Try to explain to the patient what the difficulties are and how they affect his or her activities. It may be a challenge trying to convince the patient with a right hemisphere lesion that there is a problem, because one of the common personality alterations accompanying this lesion is denial of difficulties, overconfidence, and lack of insight.

Then have the patient practice feeling walls and boundaries, thus using touch as well as vision in the process of moving around. Eliminate unnecessary furniture or decorations that may get in the patient's way. Clutter should always be avoided, both because it hampers activity and because it may cause too much sensory input and distraction for the individual. A general rule is to simplify the environment. Reduce the number of objects, noises, choices, and people. A more subdued environment permits the patient to concentrate on the task at hand with minimal distractions.

Good lighting is essential in helping to overcome these perceptual deficits. It eliminates shadows and distortions, which only complicate the problem. Bright colors on certain items may help the patient to pick out objects against a background. For example, a bright-colored bedspread against a pale wall may help the patient to determine the position of and distance to the bed.

Disturbances in depth perception cause the person to knock over glasses, cups, and other items on a food tray or overbed table. If you can teach the patient to move toward these objects very slowly and to approach them at a low level, for example at the base of a glass, you may help to cut down on accidents.

Patients who no longer understand the concepts of up and down, left and right, may need special help in self-care. If you tell the patient to put the left arm into a sleeve first, you may confuse the patient. Neither should you refer to the left arm as the "bad" arm if it is paralyzed. Rather, point to the left arm and have the patient practice putting that arm in the sleeve first. The patient who has difficulty finding the left sleeve or the top of the shirt may need to learn helpful hints such as that labels are always on the top, and perhaps to look for a special mark on the left sleeve.

One-sided neglect is also a problem that responds to nursing intervention. Again, explaining to the patient that the left side is being neglected may make the patient more aware of the problem. You can increase stimulation to that side, touching the left arm or shoulder if there is sensation, talking to the patient from the left side, and positioning the patient so that the left side is in view. Have the patient handle the ignored limbs with the other side; this action increases awareness of the neglected side. You will also have to protect the left side during activities, since the patient may not do so.

Evaluation of one-sided neglect should be carried out periodically. Assess whether the patient is using the ignored side or protecting it, handling it, or if there is greater awareness of the neglected part of the environment. If you see no improvement, you may have to try spending more time with the patient manipulating and using the left side and making the patient use it, or try attaching a small bell to the left limbs to draw attention to them.

It is difficult to help someone overcome the agnosias. You can encourage a patient to use all the senses in attempting recognition. For example, if only tactile agnosia exists, have the patient look as well as touch all items. If visual agnosia is the problem, have the patient use touch and hearing to try to identify an object or person.

Apraxia is a little easier to deal with. If a patient cannot carry out a task when asked to do so, try another approach. The person with left hemisphere damage may have difficulty understanding a verbal message anyway if there is receptive aphasia, but may be able to carry out the task if you demonstrate it first. With a right hemisphere lesion, perceptual problems may interfere with ability to learn from demonstration. These patients may be able to respond if you break the command down into simple parts. Instead of saying "Please put on your shirt," you should start with "Give me your arm. Now put it in this sleeve," etc. A combination of breaking the instructions down into small steps, using plenty of repetition and practice and giving positive reinforcement for small attempts and successes, can yield good results.

Unfortunately, we do not usually care for patients who have only perceptual problems. Most patients with brain damage severe enough to cause perceptual deficits also have problems with mobility, elimination, nutrition, or personality and intellectual changes. Some patients may have spontaneous improvement in perception; others will not. But if we give attention to perceptual deficits as well as all the other diagnoses, the patient may improve with help and practice.

SENSORY AND PERCEPTUAL DEPRIVATION

Patients who have decreased sensation and perceptual deficits are subject to sensory and perceptual deprivation. Deprivation of this type results from a decrease in sensory input, lack of variety in sensory input, and a decrease in ability to extract meaning from the input.

The causes of sensory and perceptual deprivation include not only an actual decrease in sensation, such as touch and temperature, or a decrease in vision, but also bedrest, confinement, darkness, and lack of social contact. Any patient with neurologic deficits or who is critically ill can be affected by this problem.

Symptoms of sensory and perceptual deprivation are many and varied. The patient may suddenly become irritable, restless, and confused. Extreme boredom may exist, with a decrease in attention span and sleepiness. In extreme cases there are hallucinations and delusions.

The stroke patient with homonymous hemianopsia and hemianesthesia is a candidate for deprivation. The sensory input is decreased, there may be few visitors, and if the patient is elderly, the problem is compounded. It is not unusual for these patients to become restless and have to be restrained, or to claim they see bugs on the wall and people in the windows.

Patients in intensive care units are also in danger of sensory deprivation. They are immobilized, may have decreased vision and perceptual deficits, and are surrounded by constant lights, noise, and even confusion. They are also deprived of a normal sleep cycle. Even if they are receiving sensory input, it is meaningless and monotonous. In some cases there may actually be too much of this monotonous, confusing sensory input, resulting in *sensory overload*, a related condition with symptoms like those of sensory deprivation.

Nursing Interventions

You may be able to prevent sensory and perceptual deprivation by stimulating a patient with frequent visits and conversation, touching the patient, or playing a radio or television in the room occasionally. To do much good, though, the stimulation must be meaningful for the patient. Just popping your head in the door to look at the patient or playing a radio in the room of a patient with receptive aphasia does not provide input that really enters the patient s thought process and awareness. In fact, as mentioned before, stimuli that are monotonous, unvaried, overdone, and not understood can do just as much harm as no stimuli at all.

Patients who exhibit symptoms of deprivation at night may benefit from a small light being left on. Many patients receive just enough input during the day to prevent overt symptoms, but at night, when it is dark and noise is at a minimum, the patient loses touch with the environment and displays symptoms such as confusion and climbing over the side rails.

Other interventions that may be successful include keeping familiar items from home on the patient's bedside table, encouraging phone calls, supplying the patient with his or her eyeglasses or hearing aid, and explaining various pieces of equipment in the room as well as the many hospital noises. Sensory overload can be minimized by keeping noisy machinery such as monitors and respirators as far away from the patient as possible and by keeping room lights on during the day but off or dim at night. Maintaining a normal sleep-wake cycle is very important. Try to organize your care so that the patient can have extended periods of sleep, especially at night, rather than short naps between procedures. If you follow the guideline of trying to make sensory input as normal as possible and meaningful to the patient, you can prevent many instances of sensory and perceptual deprivation.

**EXAMPLES OF NURSING DIAGNOSES RELATED
TO SENSORY AND PERCEPTUAL ALTERATIONS**

Paresthesias of lower left leg related to peripheral nerve damage; continuous burning and itching sensations.

Lack of sensation below the umbilicus related to spinal cord damage.

Loss of pain and temperature sensation on left side of body due to spinal cord trauma.

Intermittent sharp pain in the right arm related to contractures and muscle spasm.

Depression and despair related to chronic back pain.

Alterations in reading ability and self-care due to diplopia.

Potential for injury due to left visual field cut.

Alteration in spatial perception related to ambulation and self-care difficulties.

Alterations in nutrition and hygiene related to one-sided neglect.

Sensory and perceptual deprivation related to altered sensation, vision, and bedrest.

REFERENCES

Bojian, Marguerite W., and Helen M. Clark, "Counteracting Sensory Changes in the Aging," *American Journal of Nursing*, 80, no. 3 (March 1980), p. 473.

Burt, Margaret M., "Perceptual Deficits in Hemiplegia," *American Journal of Nursing*, 70, no. 5 (May 1970), p. 1026.

Conway, Barbara Lang, *Carini and Owens' Neurological and Neurosurgical Nursing*. St. Louis: The C. V. Mosby Company, 1978.

Fowler, Roy S., and Wilbert E. Fordyce, "Adapting Care for the Brain-Damaged Patient," *American Journal of Nursing*, 72, no. 10 (October 1972), p. 1832.

——, "Adapting Care for the Brain-Damaged Patient," *American Journal of Nursing*, 72, no. 11 (November 1972), p. 2056.

Gardner, Howard, *The Shattered Mind*. New York: Alfred A. Knopf Inc., 1975.

Hart, Geraldine, "Perceptual Distortion," *The Canadian Nurse*, 76, no. 5 (May 1980), p. 44.

Huston, Janet Cowan, "Overcoming the Learning Disabilities of Stroke," *Nursing 75*, 5, no. 9 (September 1975), p. 66.

Jacox, Ada K., "Assessing Pain," *American Journal of Nursing*, 79, no. 5 (May 1979), p. 895.

Johnson, Joyce H., and Maura Cryan, "Homonymous Hemianopsia: Assessment and Nursing Management," *American Journal of Nursing*, 79, no. 12 (December 1979), p. 2131.

Lamb, Sharon, "Neuroaugmentation for the Chronic Pain Patient," *Journal of Neurosurgical Nursing*, 11, no. 4 (December 1979), p. 215.

McCafferey, Margo, *Nursing Management of the Patient with Pain*, 2nd ed. New York: J. B. Lippincott Company, 1979.

——, "Relieving Pain with Noninvasive Techniques," *Nursing 80*, 10, no. 12 (December 1980), p. 55.

Norman, Susan, "Diagnostic Categories for the Patient with a Right Hemisphere Lesion," *American Journal of Nursing*, 79, no. 12 (December 1979), p. 2126.

Reinisch, Elizabeth S., "Quick Assessment of Hemiplegics' Functioning,' *American Journal of Nursing*, 81, no. 1 (January 1981), p. 102.

Roberts, Sharon L., *Behavioral Concepts and the Critically Ill Patient*, Englewood Cliffs, N.J.: Prentice-Hall, Inc., 1976.

Slater, Robert J., and Alma C. Yearwood, "MS: Facts, Faith and Hope," *American Journal of Nursing*, 80, no. 2 (February 1980), p. 276.

West, B. Anne, "Understanding Endorphins: Our Natural Pain Relief System," *Nursing 81*, 11, no. 2 (February 1981), p. 50.

9

Potential Safety Hazards

The neurologic patient is subject to many safety hazards which nurses can minimize or prevent. Protection of the patient who is ataxic or suffers from loss of balance or violent tremors or who is prone to seizures is a vital aspect of nursing care, and one that requires good judgment and forethought. This chapter deals with seizures as a major safety hazard in neurologic patient care, and with nursing interventions to protect patients who cannot protect themselves.

SEIZURES

The term *seizure disorder* is being widely used to describe a condition previously referred to as *epilepsy*: that is, a condition in which there are recurrent seizures, such as sudden attacks of muscular contractions, or abnormal autonomic function, or change in level of consciousness. There are many types of seizures and many causes. In fact, seizures are really just symptoms of underlying disease or metabolic disturbance.

Pathology

Seizures occur because of uncontrolled and excessive electrochemical impulses in the brain cells. Certain abnormal cells may emit these impulses, and may do so infrequently or frequently, sometimes causing seizures and sometimes not. The term used to describe these abnormal cells is *epileptogenic focus*, and the location of the cells is sometimes identifiable on an electroencephalogram. A localized epileptogenic focus can result from birth injuries, head trauma at any age, brain tumors, cerebral hemorrhage, or meningitis. In some cases of seizure disorders there is no known trauma or acute disease preceding the seizures, but rather the seizures result from biochemical or metabolic dysfunction, including such things as diabetes mellitus, degenerative disorders, hormonal changes, genetic defects, or nutritional deficiency. If the cause of the seizures cannot be identified, the term *idiopathic seizure disorder* (idiopathic epilepsy) is used.

Recurrent seizures will be the subject of this discussion as opposed to seizures that occur as isolated events; single or nonrecurrent seizures may occur in severely ill people whose body chemistry is abnormal, or in young children with high fevers (febrile convulsions). Recurrent seizures are often precipitated by a known event or physiologic change. Such things as lack of sleep, emotional stress, alcohol ingestion, visual stimulation, or hyperventilation may be precipitating factors. Many times, though, a specific precipitating factor for a seizure cannot be pinpointed.

Classifications of Seizures

Seizures may be either *generalized*, in which the entire brain and perhaps the entire body is affected, or they are *partial*, with only part of the brain being affected, and part of the body or general behavior and emotions showing the effects.

Generalized seizures. The disorders generally placed under this heading are grand mal (tonic-clonic) seizures, petit mal (absence) seizures, infantile spasms, myoclonic seizures, and akinetic seizures.

Grand mal seizures are those most frequently referred to as *convulsions*. They are characterized by the following sequence of events, taking place over a few minutes. The person loses consciousness and quickly goes into spasticity (tonic phase). The arms are usually flexed, the legs and neck extended. You may hear a crying sound for a few seconds as the muscles of respiration contract and force air out through narrowed airways and clenched jaws. A short period of apnea exists and may cause cyanosis until the spasticity eases and jerking movements begin (clonic phase), consisting of alternate contraction and relaxation of muscles. Increased salivation from autonomic nervous system stimulation may lead to frothing at the mouth. Urinary or bowel incontinence may also occur. Finally, the clonic movements diminish and the muscles begin to relax. After a few minutes, the person regains consciousness, but may remain confused and want to sleep.

The safety hazards involved in a generalized grand mal seizure are numerous. When the seizure begins, the person may fall and sustain an injury. During the clonic phase, there may be trauma to the head or extremities from the violent jerking movements and contact with hard objects. The tongue is frequently bitten when the jaws are clenched, and aspiration is a possibility because of the excess secretions. The most serious damage can occur if the person goes into *status epilepticus*.

Status epilepticus is a condition in which there are repeated or continuous seizures with no respite. It can occur with generalized or partial seizures, but is much more serious if generalized grand mal seizures are involved. The danger is that the brain may not receive the oxygen and glucose it needs to function and therefore suffer permanent damage. Death may occur from respiratory failure if medical treatment such as drugs, fluids, and oxygen is not instituted.

Petit mal seizures, sometimes called *absence* seizures, are usually seen only in school-aged children. Although they are generalized seizures, they are minor in effect and may not even be noticed. The child loses consciousness for just a few seconds and does not fall. If you watch closely, you may notice the attack because activity stops and there is a vacant stare. Within a few seconds the youngster resumes movement or talking and does not realize that anything has happened. Seizures may occur frequently throughout the day. Injury is not sustained in most cases.

Infantile spasms affect children in the first 2 years of life. They are generalized seizures that take rather unpredictable forms, from total body spasms to just neck spasms with or without clonic movements. They are very brief and usually cause no harm. The child may outgrow them, but many of these children are also mentally retarded and later develop other kinds of seizures.

Myoclonic seizures are one of the rarer types, characterized by brief periods of muscle contractions in the whole body or as little as one extremity. The person loses consciousness for a very short time and may fall. The contractions may be mild or violent. This disorder may occur in children or adults.

Akinetic seizures, also called *drop attacks*, are also rare, but potentially dangerous. There is a sudden loss of muscle tone and control, so sudden and without warning that the child or adult will fall and perhaps sustain injury.

Partial seizures.   This classification includes seizures that are more diverse in type and often less distinguishable as seizures because they do not involve convulsions. There are *simple partial seizures*, sometimes called *focal seizures*, in which the epileptogenic focus is probably located in the sensory or motor strip of the cerebral cortex. The person's symptoms are usually very localized motor or sensory manifestations, such as twitching of one hand or paresthesias in one arm. In some instances, simple motor seizures progress beyond one muscle group and eventually involve clonic movements of all the muscles on one side of the body. This phenomenon is known as *Jacksonian seizures*, and has even been known to progress to generalized seizure activity.

Complex partial seizures is the second grouping of partial seizures. The older term for this type is *temporal lobe epilepsy*, or *psychomotor seizures*. The epileptogenic focus has been identified in the temporal lobe. The effects of this seizure activity can be very complex. You may see automatisms such as repetitive teeth-clicking or hand-wringing or grimacing. These are unconscious acts that may be kept up for several minutes and which the person does not remember afterward. There may be sensory manifestations, such as smelling an unpleasant odor, hearing nonexistent noises, or tasting some illusory substance. The psychic elements of these seizures can also seem rather bizarre. Many victims experience intense emotions, such as anxiety and fear, distorted perception, and *déjà vu* (feeling as if something seemingly unfamiliar has been experienced before).

Complex partial seizures may be preceded by an *aura*, a warning sign that a seizure is following. Auras may be unusual sensations—visual, auditory, etc.—or feelings of dizziness or dread. It used to be thought that generalized seizures were preceded by auras, but now it is believed that some generalized seizures are preceded by complex partial seizures which take on the significance of an aura.

Consciousness may be lost during a complex partial seizure. Although the person tends to become rigid rather than falling, injuries can occur if the individual was driving or operating machinery at the time. Although the seizure lasts only a few minutes, confusion may persist for minutes or hours afterward.

Drug Therapy

The only medical treatment for seizure disorders is drug therapy. The action of *anticonvulsant* drugs is uncertain, but they seem to raise the seizure threshold by preventing normal cerebral neurons from responding to the abnormal impulses of the epileptogenic focus. About 80% of people with seizure disorders achieve satisfactory control with anticonvulsant therapy.

When therapy is begun, a drug is given until control of seizures is achieved or until toxic effects appear. Dosage may be adjusted on the basis of serum levels of the drugs. If adequate control is not obtained, a second drug is substituted or added. Your responsibility during this time is to observe for frequency and severity of seizures and for evidence of toxic or side effects.

Most anticonvulsant drugs are used to control both generalized and partial seizures, although a few are indicated for only petit mal seizures. Phenytoin (Dilantin), phenobarbital, primidone (Mysoline), and carbamazepine (Tegretol) are used for both classifications of seizures. Ethosuximide (Zarontin), trimethadione (Tridione), and clonazepam (Clonopin) are used specifically for petit mal attacks.

Side effects are common with some of the drugs and may be dangerous because of long-term therapy. Nurses play an important role in observing for side effects and teaching patients what to expect.

Phenytoin (Dilantin) is a drug frequently used for grand mal and complex partial seizures. Its side effects include gastrointestinal distress, which can be alleviated by taking it with or after meals; gingival hyperplasia (usually in children), which can sometimes be prevented by gum massage; and blood dyscrasias, necessitating periodic blood counts. Signs of toxicity from overdose are ataxia, nystagmus, and slurred speech.

Phenobarbital is also widely used for both children and adults. Its chief drawback is sedation, which can interfere with activity. However, drowsiness often decreases as the body adjusts to the drug. Virtually all the anticonvulsants are accompanied by some degree of drowsiness or dizziness, which means that the patient must have time to adjust to the drug and its effects before operating any machinery. Blood dyscrasias of one type or another are also common to these drugs, so blood work should be done at least every 6 months.

Patients who are seizure free for a few months or years may decide to try reducing the dosage of their medication or stopping it altogether to see if they can do without it. This is the most common cause of status epilepticus. If continuous seizures do develop in a noncompliant patient, they are usually treated with intravenous diazepam (Valium) and phenytoin (Dilantin).

Effects on Life Style

Seizure disorders can have widespread effects on life style. If the seizures are well controlled, these effects may be minimal, but if only partial or little control has been attained, the effects are considerable.

The person's occupation may be affected to some extent by the diagnosis of seizures. Even if satisfactory control has been attained, some employers will not permit seizure-prone employees to drive vehicles or operate machinery or engage in any work where they could be hurt or cause anyone else to be hurt. These are generally wise precautions to take, but because of these limitations, or the fear of not being hired at all, some people will not admit to their employers that they have a seizure disorder. If a person develops seizures later in life and cannot continue with an already learned occupation, some organizations, such as the Epilepsy Foundation of America, will retrain that individual for another job.

A school-aged child may face difficulties in peer relationships. No child wants to feel different from other children, but this is inevitable to some extent. The school nurse and teachers must know about the disorder and how to handle a possible seizure. Certain strenuous activities in physical education may be restricted, and even bicycle riding may be impossible unless the child is seizure free for a long period of time.

Exercise is certainly permitted, and it even helps to decrease the occurrence of seizures, but extreme exertion leading to exhaustion may be harmful. A few dangerous sports such as mountain climbing and hang-gliding are not permitted because a seizure during the progress of the sport could lead to serious injury or death. The individual should never go swimming alone because of the danger of drowning.

Driving privileges are regulated by each state. Some require the patient to report a seizure disorder; others require the physician to report it. The length of time a license is revoked for seizures also varies. Some states will grant a license if a person has been seizure free for 6 months; others require a waiting period of up to 3 years. The inability to drive may drastically affect a person's work and social life.

Alcoholic beverages are limited because they may trigger seizures in some people, and because they have a combined depressant and sedative effect when taken together with anticonvulsants. Restrictions on alcohol consumption can cause unpleasant changes in life style for many people.

One of the worst problems that seizure-disorder victims face is the social stigma of epilepsy. A significant part of the general public still has an image of an epileptic as being mentally retarded, unpredictable, and frightening. Some of these myths are being dispelled by education and the media. People with seizure disorders have the same range of IQs as the general population. It is true, however, that many people who are mentally retarded or have severe neurological disabilities also have seizure disorders. Promotion of the term *seizure disorder* rather than *epilepsy* has helped to reduce the stigma because it has a better social connotation. More education is still needed, though, to help all people realize that seizures are just a form of nervous system dysfunction, not a supernatural event or a psychotic disorder.

NURSING INTERVENTIONS IN SEIZURE DISORDERS

Nursing care of patients with seizures falls into three areas: care required during a generalized convulsive seizure, observations and assessments made during the progress of a seizure (of any kind), and patient teaching.

Care During a Convulsive Seizure

The first and most important rule in nursing a patient with seizures is that you must stay with the patient during the progress of a seizure. You may feel you want to run for help, but there is very little anyone else can do anyway. By staying with the patient you can carefully observe what is happening and protect the patient from injury.

Try to provide privacy for the patient. Seizures always draw curious onlookers. Assure other patients or visitors that everything is under control, and then close the curtain or door. If you remain calm, other people will also tend to remain under control.

If you have enough time before muscle spasticity begins and the jaws clench, insert a padded tongue blade, plastic oral airway, or folded towel between the patient's teeth. This action prevents tongue biting, but is not always possible because spasticity may occur on onset. Never try to force anything between the teeth or to pry the jaws open.

Any tight clothing around the patient's neck or chest should be loosened to prevent constriction of the airway. If there is respiratory distress or a lot of secretions, turn the patient on his or her side to allow secretions to drain, and try to extend the neck to open the airway. These last two interventions may not be possible until during or after the clonic phase.

Physical protection of the patient is also an important intervention. During the clonic phase the head may be banged against the floor, and the violent jerking movements may result in injury if the extremities hit solid objects. You can protect the head by putting a pillow under it or, if the patient is on the floor, by putting the head on your lap. Remove any objects that might cause injury. Do not try to restrain the extremities because you can do harm to bones and muscles if you try to resist the strong muscle contractions.

After the clonic movements stop, the patient may have copious amounts of secretions in the mouth and throat. If so, you may have to suction the patient. If you have previously inserted an oral airway before the teeth clenched, you can suction through it. If you inserted a tongue blade or towel at the beginning, remove it and try to suction, or insert an airway and then suction.

If the seizure does not subside within 5 minutes, you should call for help and have someone call a physician. Prolonged seizures may be the beginning of status epilepticus.

To ensure maximum protection for a seizure-prone patient, you should keep certain equipment in the room and take a few precautions. The side rails on the bed should be kept up when the patient is in bed and should be padded to prevent injury. Commercial rail pads may be available in the hospital, or you can pad the rails with bath blankets. A padded tongue blade (wrapped with gauze) and oral airway should be taped to the head of the bed where everyone can see them and they are easily accessible. A suction machine should be kept in or near the patient's room.

Temperatures should always be taken in the axilla or rectum. A nursing order as to which way the temperature is to be taken must be on the care plan. It is too dangerous to take oral temperatures, because at the start of a seizure the patient may bite and break the thermometer. Also, the patient with uncontrolled seizures should not smoke alone or take a tub bath without supervision.

Such precautions may disturb a patient who does not want anyone to know about the seizures or who cannot accept the need for special restrictions. Sitting with the patient and explaining the need for safety precautions may help to gain understanding and cooperation.

Observations During a Seizure

You may find it difficult to remember all the observations you should make about a seizure until you have seen a few. The first time or two that you observe a seizure your anxiety will be increased and may interfere with your ability to think about the things you should be observing. To overcome this problem, you should memorize a list of pertinent assessments to be made (see Table 9.1) and practice them in a role-playing situation. In a real situation, it may help you to carry a list in your pocket if you are caring for a patient with a seizure disorder.

When you become aware that seizure activity is starting, check the time. You *must* keep track of how long the entire seizure lasts as well as how long each different phase lasts. If you are observing status epilepticus, also time the intervals between seizures, if there are any.

Watch carefully to see where the abnormal movements begin. If you can determine that the seizure started in one arm or one side of the face, you may be able to help the physician determine the site of the epileptogenic focus. Also watch the eyes. If there is a localized epileptogenic focus, the eyes may move to the side away from the focus. Listen for a cry at the beginning of the tonic phase.

Then you have to continue watching the progress of muscle movements. Observe the spread of the seizure to other muscle groups or other

TABLE 9.1 Observation of a Seizure

Parameter	Observations
Time	1. Length of entire seizure
	2. Length of various phases
Movement	3. Part of body affected first
	4. Progression of movement to other parts
	5. Type of movement (spastic, clonic, tremors)
	6. Movement of eyes to one side
	7. Movement after seizure (flaccid?)
Respiratory status	8. Apnea (duration)
	9. Cyanosis
	10. Secretions (amount, color, need for suctioning)
Level of consciousness	11. Loss of consciousness or decrease in level of consciousness and duration
	12. Changes in postictal period
Pupils	13. Size
	14. Change in reactivity
Behavior	15. Automatisms
	16. Bizarre behavior
	17. Behavior in postictal period
Elimination	18. Incontinence (urine or stool)
Mouth condition	19. Postictal condition of tongue and mucous membranes (note bloody sputum)

parts of the body. Watch the movements themselves so that you will be later able to describe whether there was spasticity, clonic movements, or tremors. All these assessments may be valuable to the physician in making a medical diagnosis.

Check the pupils for size and reactivity. The pupils may dilate in a generalized seizure. Changes in pupil reaction indicate that the autonomic nervous system is involved.

Assess the patient's respiratory status. Be alert to periods of apnea and how long they last. Observe the skin or mucous membranes for cyanosis. Check secretions for color. If they are blood tinged, there may have been trauma to the tongue or oral mucosa.

The patient's level of consciousness is also important. Loss of consciousness indicates a generalized seizure, or in some cases, a complex partial seizure. Assessing changes in level of consciousness helps to determine the type of seizure. Note at what point and for how long consciousness is lost or decreased.

If there is no loss of consciousness, focus your observations on the patient's behavior. Does the patient just stand still and stare, or are there automatisms or bizarre behaviors of any kind? Describing behavior also helps the physician in arriving at a medical diagnosis.

After a seizure is over, there are assessments that you have to continue to make in the *postictal* (after the seizure) phase. Check whether the patient was incontinent of urine or stool. Both may occur in convulsive seizures, although incontinence of stool is rare. Continue observing level of consciousness until the patient is aware and can understand you, and note how long this takes.

Have the patient open the mouth so that you can inspect the tongue and mucous membranes. Injury is common in convulsive seizures, and the patient may wonder why the tongue is so sore.

Assess motor function in the postictal phase to see if there is any residual flaccidity. Assess speech for obvious changes, and note how long these changes last. Speech may be affected if the speech areas in the brain are involved. Finally, observe whether the patient goes to sleep after the seizure.

All these observations must be concisely recorded and reported after the seizure. If your observations are complete and descriptive, they can help to pinpoint the patient's problem. They will also reveal data that can help you to plan nursing care. For example, if you observe that a patient has an aura, you may be able to have the patient quickly reach a place of safety before a seizure begins. If incontinence occurs, you can plan to protect the bedding or the patient's clothing. If you discover tongue soreness, you can institute mouthwashes and get medical treatment. You will also be able to plan how to meet the patient's emotional needs after the seizure. Seizures themselves are anxiety producing and the patient may need a lot of support and comfort after a seizure episode.

Patient Teaching

To ensure patient safety and well-being after discharge from a health care facility, the patient and family must learn some basic information and safety precautions.

Enough information about seizure disorders must be given so that old myths about epilepsy are erased. The patient should know basically what is happening in the brain and what a seizure involves. You should instruct the patient to keep a record of all seizure activity. Facts such as when and how often seizures occur, what the precipitating circumstances are, what is felt and what other people observe are all helpful to the physician. The person should be warned that even though drug therapy has been started, seizures, or at least modified versions of seizures, may still occur until the dosage has been properly regulated. Of course, for a few people, drug therapy may not control seizures at all.

Information about drug therapy should be stressed. You must impress on the patient the importance of uninterrupted drug therapy, probably for the rest of his or her lifetime. Warn the patient that after being seizure free for a long time he or she will probably wonder whether the drug is still needed and may be tempted to stop taking it. Explain that stopping the drug can bring on status epilepticus.

The patient should be informed that all doctors seen need to know about the medication being taken in order to avoid drug interactions. Possible side effects of the drug should also be explained so that the patient will report them and action can be taken.

Teaching should also include instructions to carry an identification card stating the type of seizure disorder, drug or drugs being taken, physician's name, and existence of any allergies. It would be good if the person would also wear a Medic-Alert bracelet, but many people will not because they do not want to advertise their seizure disorder. Some type of medical information must be carried in case the person has a seizure when away from home. If there is prolonged postictal confusion, the person is not able to supply information even after the seizure subsides.

Instruct patients to avoid any circumstances that are known to trigger their seizures. This may include such things as alcohol consumption, fatigue, extreme exertion, emotional stress, and constipation. There are some situations that may bring on seizures but are unavoidable. This includes menstruation and febrile illnesses. Warn patients that they are more prone to seizures during this time.

The patient's family should also be taught the preceding information. In addition, parents of young children must learn how much they can let their child do, and what activities must be restricted. Tell them that it is important to let their child lead as normal a life as possible without being overprotected.

There are several community agencies that provide valuable services to people with seizure disorders. If you tell your patients that these agencies exist, they can contact them. The Epilepsy Foundation of America and the National Epilepsy League provide such services as job training, reduced prices on medications, and life insurance. The patient's social worker can be of valuable assistance in contacting these and other agencies.

You should develop a teaching plan in order to organize your content and approach to patient teaching. Teaching a seizure-prone patient does not take long, but it is very important. Evaluate the patient's and family's learning to make sure that they have grasped the material. It may be helpful to send some printed information home with the patient, especially regarding drugs, dosage schedule, side effects, and so on.

NEUROLOGIC DISORDERS THAT
PREDISPOSE TO PATIENT INJURY

Any patient with alterations of movement is subject to injury, including those with problems like spasticity, flaccidity, tremors, and ataxia. Safety precautions must be taken with patients who have multiple sclerosis, cerebral palsy, Parkinson's disease, brain damage due to trauma, and especially Huntington's disease (Huntington's chorea).

Huntington's disease is a hereditary degenerative disease of the central nervous system. It is transmitted through an autosomal dominant gene, so each child born to a person with Huntington's disease has a 50% chance of getting the disease. The pathological changes involve degeneration of the cerebral cortex and basal ganglia, usually beginning around the age of 35. The cause of such destruction is unknown. The resulting problems are deterioration of the intellect and personality, and various alterations of movement, including spasticity, choreiform movements, and rigidity, which affect ambulation, eating, and speech. The spasmotic jerking and writhing movements progress to the point where injury is common and sometimes fatal.

NURSING INTERVENTIONS TO PROTECT
INJURY-PRONE PATIENTS

Interventions to protect injury-prone patients include restraints, protective padding, use of protective headgear, and supervision in ambulation.

Restraints

Physical restraint is necessary for patients who cannot control their movements or body position, or who are not aware of danger. Although a physician's order is usually required in order to apply restraints, some institutions have policies allowing nurses to apply wrist or chest restraints independently if in their judgment they are necessary to protect the patient.

For many patients, chest restraints are adequate. For others, especially patients with extreme involuntary movements, a full torso restraint may be needed. Wrist and ankle restraints must be used with caution. They are good for protecting various tubes such as IVs, catheters, and nasogastric tubes, but they can be harmful if the patient has powerful spasms or choreiform movements. It can also be dangerous to restrain a patient who has sustained a head injury, because if he or she fights against the restraints, intracranial pressure can go up.

If you are going to get maximum protection from a restraint yet avoid injury, you have to take certain precautions. First, the restraints should be tight enough to keep the patient in the bed or chair, yet loose enough to permit a normal anatomical position and to prevent binding. If there is a possibility that a restraint strap may cause skin damage, a pad must be placed under the strap. A nursing order stating, "Release restraints and check skin condition Q2H" should appear on the care plan.

Be careful that the patient does not lie on any knots or buckles. The restraint should be tied or buckled to the bed frame or the chair frame, never to the side rails, which may be let down, and usually not *behind* a chair since many patients can reach around the chair and release them. For a patient who needs restraints but who gets too agitated when they are put on, another method of providing safety must be found. Usually, these patients require someone to stay in their room at all times.

Use of restraints should be evaluated periodically. Is the most efficient type of restraint being used? Does it allow the patient to have sufficient movement? Can the patient possibly slip out or get out of the restraint? Can the restraint be left off while someone is in the room? Without evaluation of the situation, a patient may be restrained for a longer time than necessary, or restrained more severely or less securely than is needed.

Padding

Extremely restless patients and those with violent movements may need pads on the side rails just as seizure-prone patients do. Chairs or wheelchairs may also need to be padded to prevent trauma. Foam pads, pillows, or bath blankets can be used for padding. Geriatric chairs are the best seats for patients with uncontrolled movements because they support the head against the high chair back and the tray in front also gives some support. The tray may have to be padded as well as the foot supports and any exposed metal parts around the legs.

Helmets

Uncontrolled seizures and severe ataxia may be the cause of so many falls that the danger of head injury is great. For patients with these problems, especially children, protective headgear may be the answer to preventing head injury yet not restricting activity. Figure 9.1 shows a typical protective helmet.

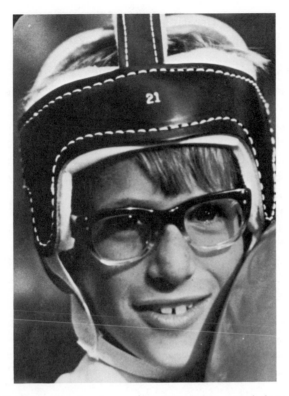

Figure 9.1 Protective headgear. (Reprinted by permission; ©J. A. Preston Corp., 1981.)

Supervised Ambulation

Many safety factors in ambulation have already been covered in Chapter 3. Some patients are prone to falls in spite of using walkers, crutches, braces, and so on. They require supervision or assistance in ambulation at all times. In addition, they should wear shoes that will not skid and that provide proper support. A waist belt or strap is a good safety measure because the assistant can pull on the belt if necessary to help the patient regain balance, or if a fall is inevitable, can lower the person gently to the floor by holding the belt.

Safety is an inherent part of all nursing care and should not be just an afterthought. Before planning any care you should consider the safety aspects of the plan and modify your approaches accordingly.

EXAMPLES OF NURSING DIAGNOSES RELATED
TO POTENTIAL SAFETY HAZARDS

Potential for physical injury due to frequent generalized seizures.

Noncompliance with anticonvulsant therapy resulting in status epilepticus.

Alterations in socialization related to seizure disorder and altered self-concept.

Lack of knowledge regarding seizures and effects on life style.

Danger of trauma related to violent muscle contractions of Huntington's disease.

Danger of falls and injury due to ataxia.

Anxiety related to fear of falling and lack of independence in ambulation.

Potential for physical injury related to use of restraints.

REFERENCES

Bruya, Margaret Auld, and Rose Homan Bolin, "Epilepsy: A Controllable Disease," *American Journal of Nursing*, 76, no. 3 (March 1976), p. 388.

Chee, Claire M., "Seizure Disorders," *Nursing Clinics of North America*, 15, no. 1 (March 1980), p. 71.

Free, Joyce W., and Carmine McPhillips, "Huntington's Disease," *RN*, 40, no. 8 (August 1977), p. 44.

Hickey, Joanne, *The Clinical Practice of Neurological and Neurosurgical Nursing*. Philadelphia: J. B. Lippincott Company, 1981.

Kukuk, Helen M., "Safety Precautions: Protecting Your Patients and Yourself," *Nursing 76*, 6, no. 6 (June 1976), p. 49.

Lovely, Mary Pat, "Identification and Treatment of Status Epilepticus," *Journal of Neurosurgical Nursing*, 12, no. 2 (June 1980), p. 93.

Misik, Irene, "About Using Restraints—with Restraint," *Nursing 81*, 11, no. 8 (August 1981), p. 50.

Norman, Susan E., and Thomas R. Browne, "Seizure Disorders," *American Journal of Nursing*, 81, no. 5 (May 1981), p. 984.

Tucker, Catherine Ann, "Complex Partial Seizures," *American Journal of Nursing*, 81, no. 5 (May 1981), p. 996.

10

Alterations in Psychosocial Functioning

Anyone who faces the prospect of acute or chronic illness is subject to stress, and behavioral responses to severe stress are inevitable. The focus of this chapter is on behavioral manifestations of illness in general, neurologic illness in particular, with attention also to the effects of sexual dysfunction due to neurologic disease. Nursing interventions for individual patients and their families will be discussed.

BEHAVIORAL MANIFESTATIONS OF ACUTE AND CHRONIC ILLNESS

The Sick Role

The person who becomes ill in American society is expected to take on the "sick role." This means that the individual relinquishes his or her usual role in society and takes on one that is compatible with illness. The sick role includes freedom from usual activities and responsibilities, increased dependency with some regression, self-concern and concern with bodily functions, and compliance with medical care. As nurses, therefore, we expect patients to be somewhat physically and emotionally dependent on us, to regress to some behaviors of an earlier developmental level, to be self-centered, and to accept docilely whatever nursing and medical care we feel the patient needs.

There are times, however, when we encounter patients who do not accept or conform to the sick role or who seem to have gone beyond their ability to cope with the stress of illness. It is not unusual to see patients with catastrophic illnesses or those facing long-term or chronic illness acting out with deviant behavior. The type and severity of illness is only one factor that can contribute to this situation. Other factors are the person's usual personality, lack of support systems, or lack of previous coping mechanisms.

The individual who has had prior personality problems will probably have even greater difficulties during illness. Impatience, selfishness, and rebelliousness are all likely to be magnified during illness. Patients who have no family, close friends, or religious ties may also have more difficulty in coping with stress. Absence of these support systems puts a great burden on the patient to handle all problems alone. Individuals who have not previously been subject to great stress may not have developed adequate coping mechanisms and find themselves in an overwhelming situation with no effective means of reducing or handling the stress. All these factors contribute to the development of deviant or extreme behaviors.

Anger

Mild expressions of anger or irritation in response to situations where needs are not being met are appropriate for anyone, well or ill. But when a rational patient becomes extremely belligerent, noncompliant, and hostile, you should begin to look for the underlying cause. Anger often results from unrelieved anxiety, frustration, forced dependency with loss of self-esteem, and perceived threats to the inner self. The patient who cannot tolerate being dependent on others or who cannot cope with the uncertainty of illness and all of the unending diagnostic tests may become angry. The patient who feels depersonalized, treated as an object in the hands of uncaring people, may become angry. The person who feels as if his or her rights have been violated and as if all control in a situation has been lost may become angry. Anger may also be seen in the patient who feels as if illness is an injustice.

Anger takes many forms of behavior. One patient may become very demanding, another very aggressive. Seductive behavior can be a sign of anger, as can constant criticism and sarcasm. You may encounter a few patients who lash out physically, as well as some who seem withdrawn. Very few patients forthrightly express their anger and the reasons for it, because they know anger is socially unacceptable, they fear retaliation, or they may honestly not know why they feel the way they do.

Depression

Transient feelings of depression during illness are expected, and are thought to be helpful in some cases, since during periods of depression the patient conserves energy. Depression that lasts for long periods of time or that interferes with recovery, however, is certainly not helpful.

Some people view depression as anger turned inward. This is a possibility that can result from any of the same causes as overt anger. Depression is often related to feelings of guilt and inferiority, and as such, may be present in patients who view sickness as punishment from God. Anyone who suffers a loss of some type, whether it be loss of a body function or loss of a particular life style, may suffer depression as a symptom of the grieving process. Being ill for a long time, or being critically ill, predisposes a patient to depression, a feeling of hopelessness, and of giving up the fight against overwhelming odds. It is not surprising that neurologic patients with disabling diseases become depressed.

How does the depressed patient appear? Any one of a number of signs may be present. Usually, the first sign is quietness, a reluctance to communicate. A person who suddenly talks less than usual may be depressed. You may observe apathy and listlessness, a lack of interest in the surroundings, and a sad appearance. The depressed person does not want to be involved in activities or take responsibility for self-care, and hygiene may suffer. Stooped shoulders, bent head, and slumped posture while in a chair could all lead you to suspect depression. The depressed patient often withdraws into a small personal world, limiting contact with the environment.

Anxiety

There are many reasons why patients become anxious, and neurologic patients, especially, often have good reason for their fears and anxieties. Just being in strange surroundings with unknown people performing intimate tasks is a threatening situation. The patient's security is further undermined by the uncertainty of the disease and its outcome, or the knowledge that great changes in life style must take place. Fear of diagnostic procedures or fear of pain or just fear of the unknown can exist. Threats to self-image and self-esteem, whether they are due to changes in appearance or inability to resume an occupation, are anxiety producing.

Anxiety may show itself in many ways. Very often, in the initial stages of hospitalization, or during the immediate time after diagnosis, denial is evident. The patient does not believe the diagnosis is true, or denies the implications of the disease or disability. During the period of denial, the person may appear happy.

Preoccupation with body functions can also be an outward sign of anxiety. Every symptom is felt, every discomfort examined, and the patient dwells on the physical functions of the body to an inordinate degree. At the same time, all the physical symptoms of anxiety, such as palpitations, gastrointestinal disturbances, anorexia, insomnia, and fatigue, may be present, and in themselves may cause the patient further anxiety. Acute anxiety can lead to outward agitation, tearfulness, or anger.

Neurologic disease may well trigger off a crisis situation in the life of a patient. The person who is faced with a difficult, anxiety-producing situation and who cannot cope with that anxiety may suffer a period of disorganization and inability to deal with life. This person needs some kind of counseling or psychiatric care to find new ways of coping and to bring in support systems. If the person in crisis receives help, successful coping and reorganization may occur, and the person becomes ultimately stronger as a result. If no help is given, that patient may continue to suffer, not only physically, but emotionally. The nurse may well be in a position to help neurologic patients in crisis.

Nursing Interventions for Deviant Behavior

Before you can intervene to help any patient with deviant behavior, you must do a full assessment of the situation and try to determine the problem that is causing such behavior. Your only source of information may be the patient, so you will have to use your knowledge of therapeutic communication to allow the patient to express thoughts and feelings that may lead you to discover the source of the problem. Therapeutic communication techniques serve a double purpose of helping you to understand the patient, and helping the patient to share feelings that have been bottled up inside.

Establishing trust.   Be prepared to spend time with the patient to establish a trusting relationship. Few patients will share their inner thoughts with a nurse they have known for only a day or two. During the time spent with this patient, show acceptance of the deviant behavior by refraining from negative comments or expressions and showing true concern for the patient's welfare.

Mobilizing support systems.   Regardless of what the deviant behavior is outwardly, the underlying cause is often fear and anxiety. So after assessing the situation, draw on whatever support systems the patient has which can help in coping with the anxiety. Include families and friends in your plans to help the patient. Try to find out what previous coping mechanisms the patient used in dealing with anxiety. Call on the clergy or anyone who can support the patient spiritually, if that will help.

Spiritual care. Studies have indicated that many patients have spiritual needs that are left unmet during illness. So include spiritual needs in your assessment. Look for cues such as Bible reading, mention of prayer or God, or fear of death. Explore such statements as "God must be punishing me" or "Why does God want me to suffer?" Offer to pray with a patient or find someone to pray with the patient if such a need is expressed. Offer to contact a clergyman, without waiting to be asked. Drawing on the strength and love of God can be a better solution for many patients than all other anxiety-reducing interventions.

Handling anger. There are several approaches you can take to help the patient who is angry. But before you can help someone who is angry, you must realize that although the anger may be directed at you, you are really not the cause and should not take it personally. Do not defend yourself, but rather allow for the expression of feelings. Let the patient know that it is acceptable to be angry and that you realize how uncomfortable it can make the patient. If the individual is behaving very aggressively or seductively, you may have to set limits on the behavior for the safety and comfort of yourself and others.

Once you have some idea of the reason for the anger, you can work to eliminate the cause or help the patient to accept the situation. For example, if the cause is that the patient believes insufficient attention is being given to his or her needs, you can discuss the situation and work out a plan of care more satisfactory to the patient and yet realistic from a nursing standpoint. If the cause is less concrete, such as the patient's belief that his or her illness is unfair and undeserved, counseling from you or the clergy or other support systems may help the patient eventually to accept the circumstances and focus on positive aspects of the situation.

If you think that you have worked out effective means of dealing with the patient's anger, you are ready to evaluate the results. Is there an overt decrease in angry behavior? Is the patient thinking rationally and in a more positive way? Is the focus of the behavior more on getting well rather than on unfounded complaints and criticisms? Does the patient verbalize greater emotional comfort and satisfaction? Positive answers to these questions confirm your belief that your interventions were appropriate and effective.

Managing depression. The depressed or withdrawn person may require different interventions. You must first try to determine whether the patient is truly depressed or only appears so because of neurologic disease such as Parkinson's disease or myasthenia gravis, which cause a masking of facial expression and sad demeanor. If through communication with the patient or family you can determine the cause of the depression, your approaches may be directed specifically at that cause. For example, if the individual is depressed because of loss of function of one arm, you can provide emotional support while helping the patient to see the potential of using the other arm for most activities.

Depressed patients should not be allowed to physically withdraw and isolate themselves from outside interests and from people. Your nursing orders should direct all nurses to encourage such patients to take responsibility for self-care and to get exercise, if possible. Include them in activities and conversation, assuming that they will take interest in what is going on. Try to give them some control over their lives by asking them to make some decisions, and then reinforce their decision with a positive attitude. Emphasize every small gain or improvement in condition or abilities. Recovery from depression can take a long time and demands the patience of everyone around the patient. If no significant progress is seen, the patient may need to be referred to a psychiatric nurse specialist or psychiatrist.

Allaying anxiety.   Anxiety is the most prevalent emotional problem among the ill, but it often responds well to nursing intervention. You can prevent a lot of anxiety by explaining patients' care to them and eliminating some of the fear of the unknown. The value of touch has long been known to reduce anxiety in many people because it gives the reassurance of not being alone or isolated.

Patients who are very agitated benefit from a structured daily schedule, because the certainty and sameness contribute to a sense of security. Having the same nurse care for the patient each day is also helpful. You should try to keep the patient's mind occupied with some type of activity and to provide physical activity. It is often helpful to reiterate to the patient your belief in his or her ability to cope with the present situation, while at the same time providing support.

Assisting in acceptance of disability.   For the patient whose disease or injury leaves permanent neurologic disability, you can assist in the achievement of emotional and intellectual acceptance of the disability. First, you can use your trusting, therapeutic relationship with the patient to help him or her realize the importance and value of continued treatment. The patient may want to give up physical or occupational therapy when only small gains are being made. If the patient trusts you, trust will also be placed in your professional judgment.

Make the most of any small improvements that you see in the patient's condition or abilities. Assist the patient to perceive even these small improvements as progress toward a goal. You can also help this person to set realistic goals to aim for in the move back toward normal living. With your greater knowledge of pathology and rehabilitation, you can tactfully tell the patient if certain goals are beyond the physical capabilities or if they are achievable goals. With your positive reinforcement, the patient will begin to feel great satisfaction from even small successes, and will not dwell as much on the limitations.

Becoming independent is an important goal for most patients and is one that may be reached with the assistance of the health team and the family. Allow your patient to be as independent as possible as soon as possible, beginning with some of the simple activities of daily living. Never keep a patient physically dependent on you because it is easier that way.

As the patient begins to face the realities of the disability and to make plans for how to return to the mainstream of living in a realistic way, achieving satisfaction and interest in life once again, you will know that acceptance of disability is developing. The patient will still have ups and downs, but will continue to progress toward a satisfactory life.

SPECIFIC EFFECTS OF NEUROLOGIC DISORDERS ON THE MIND AND EMOTIONS

The person suffering from neurologic disease or injury is subject to all the emotional hazards of general illness as well as certain effects that occur when there is damage to the nervous system.

Emotional Lability

Cerebral damage is often accompanied by emotions that fluctuate quickly from one extreme to another. The patient may be laughing one minute and crying the next. This unpredictable seesaw of emotions is termed *emotional lability*. It is commonly seen in stroke patients and may be very distressing to them, because they may be aware of it but unable to control it.

Inappropriate Behavior

Many patients who suffer hemispheric damage are left with a pattern of inappropriate behavior: that is, behavior that is incongruent with a given situation. Typical behavior may be shouting obscenities at everyone who comes in the room, throwing food off the food tray, playing with dentures, or repeatedly opening zippers. Such behavior is very embarrassing to the patient's family, especially if it occurs when visitors are around. The patient seems unaware of the meaning of such behavior and may not remember having acted in such a way if asked about it 5 minutes later.

Loss of Memory

People who have sustained cerebral damage due to stroke, trauma, surgery, or alcoholism may have a consequent memory loss. It may be a temporary loss or a permanent one, and may involve immediate recall, recent memory, or remote memory. Such a loss induces disorientation, some confusion, and perhaps a vague or specific awareness that memory has been lost.

Patients lacking immediate recall and recent memory present considerable nursing problems. They cannot retain explanations or instructions and cannot fathom where they are or who the people around them are. They are unable to function independently because they forget what they are doing before they even complete a given task.

Loss of memory may be of the *retrograde* type, meaning that events of the previous few years have been lost, but the events of the very far past are still retained. The result of this type of amnesia is that the patient tends to live in the past, as if the intervening years never occurred. Such a problem results in inevitable confusion in the present from time to time and difficulty in putting a meaningful life back together.

Loss of Abstract Thinking

Brain damage often results in the loss of ability for *abstract* thinking, leaving only *concrete* thought. This person can manipulate familiar objects correctly and can communicate about the here and now and can understand what is going on in a familiar situation. The difficulty arises when faced with an unfamiliar situation or with conversation that deals with concepts and ideas rather than concrete things. Such a person cannot interpret a saying such as "A bird in hand is worth two in the bush," and cannot use problem-solving methods to arrive at a decision by weighing ideas.

The implications that loss of abstract thinking has for the social relations of the affected individual are tremendous. The inability to make more than routine decisions or judgments, the loss of true conversational abilities, the loss of interpretive abilities, and the loss of a sense of humor force this person into a very limited, dependent life style. The saddest thing is that victims of such a disability may be aware of their problem and grieve over it, yet not have the mental capabilities to understand what has really happened.

Effects of Frontal Lobe Damage

Trauma, especially penetrating trauma, to the frontal lobes of the brain causes unique effects on the personality. There is loss of motivation, enthusiasm, goal setting, and concentration powers. The person loses some of the social graces, appreciation of neatness and hygiene, and knowledge of appropriate behavior for a given social setting. In general, there is apparent lack of concern about accomplishments and lack of direction in life, yet the pure intellect is hardly touched. Although this person may be physically and intellectually capable of resuming a job and productive life, he or she is unlikely to do so.

Confusion

Confusion is not necessarily a neurologic problem, but can result from many metabolic and psychological states. Brain damage is, however, one of the leading causes of confusion, whether it is temporary or permanent. After severe head injuries, confusion accompanied by very restless or hostile behavior is common. Many patients who are slowly recovering from coma exhibit this type of overactive behavior which may last for days or weeks.

The confused patient's mind is not working with clear and organized thoughts. On the contrary, thoughts are disorganized and incongruent with reality. Family members and friends may appear to be strangers, the environment may seem threatening, and circumstances are not understood. Stimuli are often misinterpreted. For example, abdominal pain due to intestinal gas may be interpreted as pain from being hit by one of the strangers in the room.

It is not surprising that the confused patient sometimes shows paranoid tendencies. Since no sense can be made of the environment, the person struggles to find a reason for the frightening or painful experiences that are taking place. The only reason which seems to present itself is that someone is attempting some kind of harm. The person may be aware enough to know that other people in the environment are in control, and these are the people who are feared. This type of patient usually rejects all reassurances that no one has meant any harm.

Any confused patient may give evidence of having delusions and hallucinations. There may be visual or auditory hallucinations, with the patient seeing or hearing things that do not exist. Delusions such as believing that the hospital room is a prison cell, or that hospital food has been cooked by a family member, occur. Again, the patient is trying to make sense of the frightening environment.

Confabulation is a phenomenon exhibited by many people in a confused state. If you ask a confused patient to explain why he or she is in the hospital you may get an answer like "I just came to visit my nephew Henry, who has been sick." Making up stories and explanations is not done in a lying sense, but is the patient's honest attempt to reason through the situation and explain what is going on. Usually, the confabulations have some grain of truth in them.

Nursing Interventions

The nurse can help the patient who has sustained brain injury to control emotions and behavior, make sense of the world, and to reestablish mental stability. It is the nurse who spends the most time with the patient and who can best assess behavior patterns and find approaches that work for a particular patient.

Minimizing emotional lability.   Patients afflicted with emotional lability need assistance in controlling the wide swings of emotional response. If your patient who has been very quiet and somewhat depressed starts laughing inappropriately, you can try interrupting the laughter by talking about something else, and allow the patient a little time to regain control. Snapping your fingers may be enough to stop uncontrolled crying or moaning. You may choose to mention the incident to the patient and say that you understand that such outbursts are not under the patient's control. If you find a means of stopping the crying or laughing, write a nursing order explaining how to proceed. For example, "If crying begins without apparent cause, clap your hands in front of the patient's face to stop the crying."

Coping with inappropriate behavior.   For those patients who behave inappropriately and do not realize they are doing so, and who cannot remember doing so even when it is pointed out to them, there is little we can do. But some people with hemispheric damage and inappropriate behavior *do* respond to nursing action. As soon as the behavior has taken place, comment on it, letting the patient know it was not a good way to act and that there is a better way. For example, if your patient throws potatoes off the food tray, say something like, "You have made a mess on the floor. If you don't like the potatoes, just push them to the side." The patient may get the idea and correct the behavior. If so, praise the appropriate behavior. Do not keep reprimanding the patient or harping on the problem. If one comment does not work, let it go and try again at a later time.

Compensating for memory loss.   Loss of memory is a problem that requires delicate nursing care. If the patient lacks immediate recall and recent memory, you may have to serve as the patient's memory and help the patient use memory devices. Since this person probably forgets names and facts soon after you supply them, you will have to repeatedly give the same information without showing impatience. Repeat your name every time you enter the room. Tell the patient exactly what you are there for, even though you may have explained it only a short time before. You may give the patient a schedule or chart of the daily routine to help explain what is going on and to serve as a reminder. Instructions will have to be written out if you expect them to be followed when you are not with the patient.

If the patient is disturbed by the inability to remember or retain information, give the reassurance that you are there to help with remembering and to make sure that important things get done. In cases where remote memory has been lost, fill in the gaps for the patient as best you can when the patient requests the information.

Dealing with loss of abstract thinking.   When a patient has lost the ability to think abstractly, you cannot restore that ability. But you can improve communication and help make the patient feel more comfortable in the situation. Since the patient thinks in concrete terms, use concrete terms in talking to the patient and in making explanations. Do not say, "Mr. Jones, I want you to get more exercise" but rather, "Mr. Jones, I'm going to take you for a walk around the bed." Make conversation about everyday things that are familiar to the patient.

Do not expect Mr. Jones to make any complex decisions or come up with solutions to problems. If you want him to choose his own clothing for the day, do not say, "Mr. Jones, what do you want to wear today?" but instead, hold up two pairs of pajamas and ask him to choose between the two. Avoid the use of humor, since the patient may not understand your meaning and may misinterpret what you say.

Assisting the patient with frontal lobe damage.   There is not a great deal that the nurse can do to improve the functioning of a patient who has permanent damage to the frontal lobes of the brain. Apathy, flat affect, and inattention to socialization are part of the new personality. Rather than let the person withdraw or lose all interest in life, however, you should encourage good hygiene and a neat appearance, encourage the patient to talk to you, and try to foster interest in some group activities. Enlist the help of the family in socializing with the patient. Many such brain-damaged people are found in long-term-care facilities, where group activities may be provided.

Helping the confused patient. Unfortunately, one of the most effective nursing interventions that nurses ever use, therapeutic communication, may not work with a confused patient. You cannot use this means of eliciting thoughts and feelings, defining goals, and working through problems, because you cannot reach the person through rational thought. So you will be forced to fall back on less sophisticated means to help make the confused patient feel more comfortable and deal with the world more successfully.

Your first goal should be to make the patient's environment less strange and frightening. Repeatedly orient the patient to the room or the unit, to the time, the circumstances, and the people the patient will be seeing. Surround the patient with familiar belongings, if possible. Objects from home may help the patient to make contact with reality and may serve as a source of security.

Try to spend enough time with the person so that you become a familiar and friendly face. When you talk, place yourself on a level with the patient's eyes and try to maintain eye contact. Explain everything that you are doing right before you do it. Warn the patient if what you are doing is going to cause discomfort. Constant explanations and preparation may cut down on persecution delusions and paranoid feelings. Even if the patient does accuse you of some type of persecution, remain pleasant and kind and say, "It must be terrible to feel that people here are hurting you." Eventually, your kind manner may begin to speak to the patient.

Avoid going along with a patient's delusions and hallucinations. You should not say that you see the spiders on the wall if they aren't there or that you hear "Mother" calling if it is not true. Just say, "I know you think you see spiders, but I don't see any." Then go on to talk about a subject that will help to orient the patient.

Confusion combined with extreme restlessness and hostility is a difficult situation to handle. A patient may have to be restrained if he or she is pulling on tubes or climbing out of bed or trying to hurt others. Restraints should be applied only when absolutely necessary. Some patients become even more restless and agitated when restrained, and instead may have to have someone present at all times for protection and to provide a calm and reassuring environment.

When you find some successful approaches for dealing with confusion in your patient, make sure to document them. Revise your care plan as necessary to eliminate unhelpful interventions and include new interventions that work.

ALTERATIONS IN SEXUALITY
DUE TO NEUROLOGIC DISORDERS

A person's sexuality is made up of many factors, such as body image, self-esteem, sex role, need for intimacy, and moral values, as well as performance of sexual activity. All of these aspects can be affected directly or indirectly by neurologic disorders or disability.

Paralysis, paresis, deformity, and tremors all make an impact on an individual's self-image or body image. When body image is affected, the person begins to doubt his or her attractiveness to the opposite sex and desirability as a mate.

Disability brings changes in life roles and sometimes sex roles, with husbands becoming the financially dependent partner or wives having to give up the usually performed roles and take on new ones. Adolescents and young adults just achieving independence and establishing satisfying relationships with members of the opposite sex may be forced to become dependent again on parents. These changes in roles have an impact on sexuality.

If a married person becomes disabled, there is fear of not being able to satisfy the partner's sexual needs or of being repugnant to the spouse. A marriage that has been on shaky ground prior to the disability may not be able to withstand the pressures of chronic illness or changed life style.

An unmarried person who becomes disabled may fear never finding a mate, or of finding someone to love but being unable to meet all the demands of marriage. There may be anxiety due to lack of information about sexual functioning and how it is affected by disability.

In some cases, sexual desire may be diminished if there is chronic fatigue, weakness, or painful spasticity. This decrease in libido may foster guilt, or place new stress on a relationship.

Pathophysiology That Affects Sexual Functioning

Paralysis and weakness. Paralysis and weakness may both interfere with sexual functioning in people with spinal cord injury, multiple sclerosis, myasthenia gravis, and stroke, as well as many related conditions. Muscle weakness and fatigue make sexual activity difficult. Paralysis may make certain coital positions impossible. In men, the most devastating effect of these problems is on the ability to have or maintain erections.

Spinal cord-injured males vary greatly in their ability to have erections. Those with upper motor neuron damage have a high percentage of reflexogenic erections, that is, erections that are stimulated physically.

The incidence of psychogenic erections, those stimulated by thought or emotion, is low in these men. In the case of lower motor neuron lesions, the incidence of psychogenic erections is higher, and reflexogenic rather low.

The *extent* of the lesion is just as important in predicting ability as is the *level* of the lesion. Complete lesions, such as complete transection of the cord, have a poorer sexual prognosis than do incomplete lesions. Varying statistics have been published about erectile ability with various types of lesions, as reported by spinal cord-injured males. However, overall statistics vary greatly; anywhere from 50 to 90% of these men report erections of some type, depending on which study you read. It is important to realize that although the man may have some erectile function, that does not mean that he necessarily has complete or sustained erections necessary for intercourse. It seems safe to say that only about 20% of spinal cord-injured males have adequate erections.

Men with multiple sclerosis have many similar problems. The major difference, though, is that multiple sclerosis is characterized by remissions and exacerbations, making sexual functioning unpredictable. Very often after an exacerbation with paralysis or weakness that interferes with erections, the man with MS may continue to have sexual difficulties, even during remission. This continued effect may be psychological in origin.

Females with paralysis or weakness also have problems with sexual function, but since the female role is physiologically more passive, they can still participate in intercourse, although perhaps with less pleasure. Women are affected more by problems of sensation.

Loss of sensation.   Since sensation is such an important part of sexual relations, loss of sensation can have severe effects on sexual function and sexual enjoyment. Complete spinal cord lesions usually result in loss of pelvic sensation in men and women. Incomplete lesions have unpredictable effects on sensation. Multiple sclerosis may also interfere with pelvic sensation. A combination of impaired sensation and impaired pelvic vasocongestion can cause a lack of orgasm in males and females. Lack of sensation other than in the pelvic area can also affect sexuality. The quadriplegic who has no sensation below the shoulders is deprived of tactile stimulation almost completely.

Fertility and infertility.   Neurologic disease or injury does not usually affect female fertility or the ability to deliver a child normally, unless there has been damage to the pituitary gland. Transient hormonal imbalances are seen after neurologic trauma, but they usually subside without treatment. After spinal cord injury, menstruation stops for a few months but then returns to normal. Conception presents no difficulties, and normal vaginal deliveries can take place even in quadriplegics.

The fertility statistics are quite different for men with neurologic disability, however. There is a high incidence of sterility in men with spinal cord injury or damage to the pelvic nerves. Sterility can be a result of hormone imbalance, impaired temperature levels in the scrotum affecting spermatogenesis, or impaired ejaculation. Many neurologically impaired men have retrograde ejaculation, in which semen is propelled backward into the bladder rather than emptying through the urethra.

Spasticity. In only a few cases is spasticity a deterrant to intercourse. Severe spasticity in cerebral palsy or other upper motor neuron disability with adductor spasms could create a problem, but can usually be controlled by medication.

Incontinence. Urinary or bowel incontinence can be a very embarrassing occurrence during sexual activity and can interfere both physically and psychologically with function and libido. Emptying the bladder or bowel before sexual activity can help to prevent the problem. An indwelling catheter can be removed prior to intercourse and reinserted soon after, or can be left in place. A man can fold and tape his catheter back along the penis and cover it with a condom; a woman can tape the catheter to one side. Good hygienic practices are necessary to prevent transmission of chronic urinary infections.

Nursing Interventions

The primary role of the nurse in alleviating problems related to sexuality is to be willing to listen to and discuss the patient's concerns. Modesty or embarrassment may make the patient unwilling to bring up the subject, so the nurse should give a broad opening statement which allows the patient the freedom to speak. Saying something such as "A lot of people with your problem wonder about their future sex lives" gives the patient a chance to ask questions and admit to worries.

The nurse must already have established a helpful trusting relationship with the patient before broaching a subject like this. Even if the patient feels comfortable with the nurse, he or she may not be able to talk about sexual concerns because of ingrained reticence and embarrassment. During the course of the patient's hospitalization, only one nurse or physician should be designated to assess and intervene in matters relating to sexuality. The patient should not have to expose such private matters to every health care worker that comes along.

The physician may be the person to discuss the physiologic aspects of sexual functioning with the patient. An in-depth knowledge of the patient's pathology may be needed to predict future function. The physician is often the best person to discuss treatments such as penile implants for impotence or artificial insemination as a means of having a family.

There are many aspects of sexuality that do fall within the realm of counseling by nurses. You can follow up after the physician has talked to the patient and find out if there are further questions or misunderstandings. With even a basic knowledge of sexual physiology, you can answer many of the patient's questions. Counseling may encompass the whole topic of intimacy versus sex. The disabled person must begin to realize that impotence or lack of sensation do not mean the end of a sex life. Establishing an intimate caring relationship with another person involves far more than just intercourse, and alternative ways can be found of pleasing a loved one and meeting each other's needs.

You must avoid the danger of being overly optimistic in regard to the patient's future sexual functioning and satisfaction. Not every disabled person will achieve or regain a satisfactory sex life, but with time and counseling, many will adjust to living with the disability, even in this regard. If it becomes apparent that your counseling is not helping the patient adequately, that sexual concerns are increasing or are hampering other aspects of rehabilitation, it may be necessary to initiate a referral to a psychiatrist, clergyman, or social worker who can assist the patient.

ASSISTING FAMILIES OF PATIENTS WITH NEUROLOGIC DISORDERS

Family Reactions

During the period of acute or critical illness, after the diagnosis or occurrence of injury to the patient, the family will experience some fairly predictable reactions. Shock and disbelief may be the first reaction. The mind cannot yet adjust to the rapid change in circumstances and the overwhelming reality. When the feelings of unreality begin to dissipate, acute anxiety may be felt. If the patient is in a critical care facility, this fact may spell impending death to the family. The complicated machinery around the bedside is intimidating and threatening. The family is too anxious to be able to absorb everything they are being told, and may be unable to comprehend terms being used, yet be afraid to ask questions.

Anxiety may be followed by anger or depression with feelings of helplessness. The family members, who are usually a source of support to each other, may not be able to feel that support any longer. If the patient is usually the strongest support, the family may be floundering. If the other family members are the stronger supporters, they may feel helpless at being unable to assist the patient because of separation during hospitalization.

Feelings of guilt often assail the family. Parents may feel they did not care for their child well enough. Spouses may feel guilty because of a recent argument or denial of the patient's illness. Guilt may also result if the family feel they are not helping the patient in any way, or if they are unable to visit very often.

Following the acute stage of illness, some problems may resolve themselves and new problems may appear. When it becomes evident that the patient may have permanent disabilities, the family may again feel unable to cope. They may be bewildered by changes in the patient's behavior or personality. They may be ashamed of their loved one, who was once a capable person but who is now confused or shouting obscenities or drooling or incontinent.

Economic concerns may begin to come under consideration. Lengthy hospitalization or rehabilitation is costly, even if the family has medical insurance. Home care or home alterations may also be a financial drain. If there is no extended family to help, economic burdens may begin to affect relationships and interfere with recovery of the patient.

Nursing Support

The nurse can serve as a source of support to both the patient and family. Listen to what the family is saying and watch how they are reacting. Encourage them to talk about their feelings and assure them that they are responding normally in a difficult situation. Explain the various aspects of the patient's care, including simple explanations of the equipment in the room. Assure them that much of the care is routine and is designed to monitor the patient's condition and does not necessarily indicate that the patient's condition is grave.

Try to spend at least a few minutes with the family each day, outside the patient's room if possible. Talk about progress that the patient has made and answer any questions that you can. It may help the family to get involved in the patient's care. Find out if feeding the loved one or helping with positioning or bedmaking would make the family feel better, but be careful that you do not push the family into activities they are reluctant to take on. If they do want to take part in the patient's care, work with them closely until they feel secure in the situation. Indicate in your nursing orders which aspect of care the family will be involved in. Orders such as "Position patient in semi-Fowler's at 11:45 so family can feed lunch at 12:00" or "Teach wife how to record fluids on the I&O sheet" will make clear to all the staff just how much care the family will carry out.

When it is time to begin activating discharge plans, start to prepare the family. You may have to teach them how to care for the patient or how to assist with care. The family should feel secure and competent with all procedures before the patient is discharged. Sending the patient home for a weekend before the actual discharge date is helpful in getting the family to see any deficiencies in their abilities or any practical problems they may encounter in the home.

It is a natural reaction for loving families to want to overprotect a disabled loved one. Unfortunately, this reaction often causes undue dependency and failure to resume any kind of normal life. While working with the family, you should stress the fact that the patient must be allowed to achieve as much independence as possible. If the family members see you placing certain expectations on the patient, and see the patient achieving them, they will realize that the patient does have many capabilities as well as disabilities.

Disabilities and handicaps that prevent an individual from resuming a previous occupation or role do not preclude taking on new activities or roles. In your counseling with the family, encourage them to help the patient find useful things to do, activities that help the family and give meaning to life.

Economic problems can be referred to a social worker who has the most information about insurance coverage, rehabilitation centers, community resources, and vocational training. The social worker or discharge planner will also be very involved if it becomes necessary to have the patient transferred to a nursing home or other long-term institutional setting. The family that cannot care for their loved one at home and must arrange for institutionalization also needs your support. They often seek the nurse's advice and reassurance that they are doing the right thing for their loved one. By guiding them and supporting them at such a time, you may help to prevent future guilt about the decision they have made.

Helping your patient's family can be a very rewarding experience. It may be emotionally draining to try to cope with distraught family members, but when you see them responding to your support and concern, you will feel repaid many times over.

**EXAMPLES OF NURSING DIAGNOSES RELATED
TO PSYCHOSOCIAL ALTERATIONS**

Anxiety related to dependence and loss of control.

Noncompliance with nursing regimens related to feelings of depersonalization.

Maladaptive coping patterns related to long-standing personality disorder.

Depression related to loss of many body functions.

Maladaptive coping patterns related to preoccupation with physical symptoms.

Emotional lability related to brain damage; cries uncontrollably without apparent reason.

Potential for injury due to short attention span.

Anxiety related to memory loss.

Confusion related to brain damage; is disoriented to time, place, and person.

Alteration in sexuality; fears being unable to maintain a satisfactory sex life.

Anxiety related to fear of infertility.

Ineffective family coping; daughter states that necessary home functions are not being carried out.

Ineffective family coping related to mother's guilt over accident.

REFERENCES

Baxter, Robert T., and Alan Linn, "Sex Counseling and the SCI Patient," *Nursing 78*, 8, no. 9 (September 1978), p. 46.

Beland, Irene L., and Joyce Y. Passos, *Clinical Nursing, Pathophysiological and Psychosocial Approaches*, 3rd ed. New York: MacMillan Publishing Co., Inc., 1975.

Fish, Sharon, and Judith Allen Shelly, *Spiritual Care: The Nurse's Role*. Downers Grove, Ill.: Inter-Varsity Press, 1978.

Fowler, Roy S., and Wilbert Fordyce, "Adapting Care for the Brain-Damaged Patient," *American Journal of Nursing*, 72, no. 11 (November 1972), p. 2056.

Kolodny, Robert, William H. Masters, Virginia E. Johnson, and Mae A. Biggs, *Textbook of Human Sexuality for Nurses*. Boston: Little, Brown and Company, 1979.

McDonnell, Margaret, and others, "MS Problem Oriented Nursing Care Plans," *American Journal of Nursing*, 80, no. 2 (February 1980), p. 292.

Moritz, Derry Ann, "Understanding Anger," *American Journal of Nursing*, 78, no. 1 (January 1978), p. 81.

Nicksic, Esther, "Problem Patients or Problem Nurses?" *Nursing Outlook*, 29, no. 5 (May 1981), p. 317.

Roberts, Sharon, *Behavioral Concepts and the Critically Ill Patient*. Englewood Cliffs, N.J.: Prentice-Hall, Inc., 1976.

Stryker, Ruth Perin, *Rehabilitative Aspects of Acute and Chronic Nursing Care*. Philadelphia: W. B. Saunders Company, 1972.

Taylor, Joyce W., and Sally Ballenger, *Neurological Dysfunctions and Nursing Intervention*. New York: McGraw-Hill Book Company, 1980.

Trockman, Gordon, "Caring for the Confused or Delirious Patient," *American Journal of Nursing*, 78, no. 9 (September 1978), p. 1495.

Walke, Mary Anne Kelly, "When a Patient Needs to Unburden His Feelings," *American Journal of Nursing*, 77, no. 7 (July 1977), p. 1164.

Wu, Ruth, *Behavior and Illness*. Englewood Cliffs, N.J.: Prentice-Hall, Inc., 1973.

11

Neurologic Alterations
in Children

Most of the information in the preceding chapters can be applied to children with neurologic problems. However, there are some variations in assessment and interventions that are required because of the unique aspects of neurologic disease that can be found in children, and because a nurse's approach to a child patient must be guided by growth and development factors. How neurologic assessment differs for children will be discussed first, followed by the most common pediatric neurologic problems and nursing interventions.

NEUROLOGIC ASSESSMENT OF A CHILD

The actual assessment process of checking level of consciousness, awareness, pupil response, vision, vital signs, and motor and sensory function is basically the same for both children and adults (see Chapter 2). What differs, though, is the comparison of findings to what is normal for a particular child's stage of growth and development, and the approach you would use to communicate with the child. First, you must have a basic knowledge of growth and development, especially as it relates to motor development, reflexes, changes in vision, and intellectual development. Second, you must be able to talk to a child on his or her level, knowing what that age group is generally capable of understanding, what kinds of responses and behaviors may be expected, and what interests the child might have. If you communicate with a child in the appropriate manner, your chances of obtaining correct information and accurate results are greatly increased. Following are assessments or considerations in the assessment process that pertain particularly to children.

Mental Status

Level of consciousness.   The same terms used to describe level of consciousness in adults can be applied to children, such as awake, lethargic, stuporous, comatose. A description of the exact behavior of the child means more than just using a label, though. Be aware that children are often harder to arouse from sleep than are adults, and may require much greater stimulation to waken them. You must be careful to differentiate between a very sound sleep and unconsciousness. Children also take longer to reach complete wakefulness and should not be assessed until they have been awake for a while.

Degree of awareness.   To check the child's degree of awareness, you must ask questions that reveal whether the child is aware of time and place. But a preschool child may not be aware of the time of day or remember the name of a town or hospital. It might be better to ask a preschooler his or her name. After age 4 a child should remember both first and last names.

Memory is also an age-related function and should be assessed with developmental stages in mind. *Immediate recall* in an adult is considered satisfactory if the adult can repeat a series of five or six numbers after you have said them. A child younger than 4 years old probably cannot be tested this way. Between 4 and 6 years old the child can be expected to remember three numbers and after 6 years old, five numbers.

Recent memory should be evaluated in a preschool child by showing a familiar object, then hiding it and after a few minutes asking the child what the object was. A school-aged child can be asked similar questions to those asked of an adult, such as "What did you eat for breakfast?"

Remote memory is tested in the adult by asking about things that happened years ago. But for a child, the far past may be the previous day, and for a preschool or young school-aged child an appropriate question might be, "What color shirt were you wearing yesterday?" or 'What did you do before you went to bed last night?"

Language comprehension will of course vary with developmental level. It may be difficult to assess comprehension in a toddler, because if you give a command, even if there is comprehension, the child may be unwilling to obey. You may have to rely on the mother to tell you about recent language comprehension. Older children can be given simple commands such as "Close your eyes" to see if they understand and follow directions.

Pupils

The pupillary reflex is present at birth, so pupils should constrict on a flashlight check at any age. However, infants have rather small pupils to begin with, and it may be difficult to see constriction occur. You must be sure to check pupils in a darkened room so that they are as dilated as possible before testing.

Vision

To test gross visual abilities, you must know age-related norms. An infant can see objects within about a 3-foot range and the eyes will follow an object for a short distance. You can test vision by holding a bright-colored toy about 2 feet away from the infant and watching the eyes. By 3 years old, a child can follow the directions associated with an E chart. By school age, a Snellen chart can be used. Visual fields can be tested in the school-aged child in the same manner as is used for adults.

Motor Function

Muscle strength and tone should be assessed the same way it is done for the adult. Knowledge of the development of motor function is also essential. Developmental milestones between the activity of a newborn who can only lift the head off the bed, to a preschooler whose gross motor abilities are close to that of an adult, should be understood. Whatever age child you are evaluating, you must know what the expected motor abilities are.

A 2- or 3-month-old child should be able to lift both head and chest off the mattress and by 4 or 5 months the child should be able to roll over. Between 6 and 8 months, sitting unsupported should be possible; by 9 months old most children can pull themselves to a standing position. By 14 months, all children should be capable of standing alone and walking. The greater coordination required to walk up steps independently may not be achieved until almost 2 years of age.

Reflexes

There are many reflexes present in the newborn and many that develop during infancy. They usually reflect the immaturity of the nervous system and they disappear as the nervous system develops. Failure of newborn reflexes to disappear within a certain time frame may indicate the presence of a neurologic disorder. Similarly, failure of other reflexes to appear at certain intervals during infancy may also lead to the suspicion of pathology. Reflexes that are too strong or too weak or which are present on only one side of the body also indicate neurologic impairment. Some of the commonly elicited reflexes will be discussed.

The *rooting reflex* is stimulated when something touches the infant's cheek; the baby turns its head toward that side, looking for food. This reflex should diminish in about 3 or 4 months. The *sucking reflex* occurs when the baby's lips are touched. The sucking motion that is stimulated serves to allow the infant to suck from a nipple; it should disappear around 6 months. Abnormalities in the rooting and sucking reflexes may reveal extensive neurologic dysfunction.

The *extrusion reflex* is one in which the infant will push out any food placed on the front of the tongue. It is a protective mechanism to prevent a baby from swallowing foreign objects. It diminishes at about 4 months old.

The *palmar grasp* (see Figure 11.1) reflex lasts until about 6 months. It involves the infant grasping anything placed in the palm of the hand. The *plantar grasp* reflex involves the same action in the foot, with the toes doing the grasping. It disappears by the end of one year when the child is ready to stand. If either of these reflexes persist for an unusually long time, the suspicion of cerebral palsy exists.

The *Moro reflex* is stimulated by loud noise or sudden movement. The infant at first extends both arms and legs (see Figure 11.2), the arms looking as if they are about to embrace something. Then the arms and legs are drawn up against the body. This is a protective reflex that gets progressively weaker as the baby matures. If it persists beyond 9 months. the child may have a neurologic disorder.

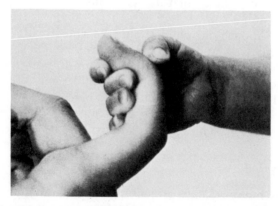

Figure 11.1 The palmar grasp reflex. (Courtesy of Mead Johnson and Co., Evansville, Ind.)

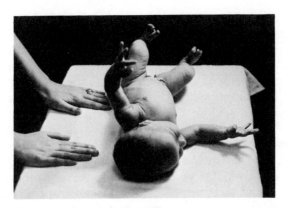

Figure 11.2 The Moro reflex. (Courtesy of Mead Johnson and Co., Evansville, Ind.)

The *tonic neck* reflex is exhibited when the infant lies on the back with the head turned to one side. The arm and leg on the side toward which the head is turned extend, and the other arm and leg flex (see Figure 11.3). This reflex usually disappears by the time the baby is 3

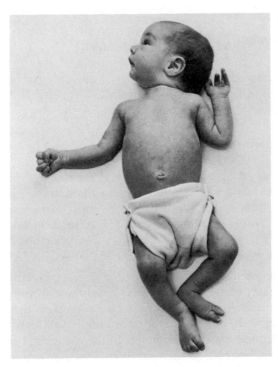

Figure 11.3 The tonic neck reflex. (Courtesy of Mead Johnson and Co., Evansville, Ind.)

months old. If it still exists well beyond that age, neurologic damage, especially cerebral palsy, is suspect.

The *Landau reflex* is acquired at about the age of 3 months and lasts up to 2 years. If, while the infant is in prone position you hold his or her trunk in the palm of your hand and lift the trunk off the mattress, the head and legs should extend. If you flex the head, the legs and arms should also go into flexion. Failure of this reflex to appear reveals motor weakness.

The *parachute reflex* begins between 6 and 9 months of age. The infant is held, face down over a table, but suspended in the air by your hands under the trunk. If you suddenly lower your hands, the baby's arms should extend as if in protection. Delayed appearance of this reflex response may be due to neurologic deficits. An extreme flexion response may indicate cerebral palsy.

Whether you test for these reflexes yourself or read the findings on the physician's history and physical sheet, you should be familiar with the significance of these major reflexes at various ages. With a basic knowledge of neurologic assessment of a child, you can begin to plan care based on the child's capabilities and physical condition.

COMMON PEDIATRIC NEUROLOGIC PROBLEMS

The most common and most profound neurologic problems seen in infants and children will be discussed, relating the altered body functions to the pathology.

Spinal Cord and Cerebral Damage

The effects of spinal cord and cerebral damage on children and adults is similar, but certain unique conditions do occur in children. For example, in infants spinal cord damage is most often caused by myelomeningocele. Cerebral damage may be due to birth injury, falls, or from parental abuse.

Myelomeningocele. A myelomeningocele is a congenital defect in the lumbosacral spine, consisting of incomplete fusion of one or more vertebral arches (spina bifida), herniation of the meninges through the spinal defect (meningocele), and protrusion of the spinal cord itself into the external sac formed by the meninges. Since the spinal cord ends at the level of the myelomeningocele, paralysis and sensory loss will be in a similar pattern to that seen in any spinal cord damage (see Chapter 3).

The lesion is usually in the lumbosacral area, so many of these children, if they live past the first few months, will be able to ambulate with braces and crutches.

Bowel and bladder elimination is affected in almost all of these cases, and either constipation or fecal incontinence may occur. Neurogenic bladder is of the lower motor neuron type (see Chapter 4). Sexual functioning is bound to be affected in some way. Although secondary sex characteristics develop normally, sexual functioning in males will be affected by the spinal cord defect. Social relationships with the opposite sex may be hampered by disability.

Head injury. Cerebral trauma manifests itself differently in children from in adults. Since cerebral structures are more pliable in children, they may "give" more when the head is struck, and less damage will be sustained than in an adult. However, some tissues are thinner in children (especially in premature infants) and are more prone to tearing and rupture. Children heal faster than adults and usually recuperate faster from stressful and traumatic situations. Infants and young children may not show as many signs of neurologic disturbance, because of the immaturity of the nervous system and the ability of the skull to expand and accommodate swelling.

Injury to the head may be sustained during the birth process, especially during difficult deliveries where there is cephalopelvic disproportion, or where forceps are required. In young children, falls are a frequent cause of head injury. Falls from a bassinet, crib, or later from skates and monkey bars often involve trauma to the head. Children of any age may receive head injuries from abusive parents. Direct blows to the head or blows that cause a fall are common in child abuse cases and may be repeated several times before the problem is discovered.

Frequently seen effects of head injury are *cerebral concussion, contusion, laceration, subdural hematoma,* and *subarachnoid bleeding* Cerebral concussion involves a shifting of the brain with no bleeding or permanent damage. The child loses consciousness or has a noticeable decrease in the level of consciousness for at least a few minutes.

A subdural hematoma is a collection of blood between the dura and arachnoid. It can develop rapidly within 24 hours or slowly over a period of weeks. Subarachnoid bleeding occurs in the subarachnoid space, and both types of bleeding can result in symptoms of increased intracranial pressure.

Cerebral contusion and laceration are very serious and potentially life-threatening conditions. There is bleeding within the cerebral tissues and edema also occurs. Again, this can lead to increased intracranial pressure.

Increased Intracranial Pressure

Elevated pressure in infants and children can be caused by head injury, as just mentioned, or by *hydrocephalus* which is the accumulation of abnormally large amounts of cerebrospinal fluid in the ventricles of the brain leading to an enlarged head or increasing intracranial pressure. The pathology exists either in the ventricles or in the passages between them, where an obstruction causes the CSF to acccumulate, or in the subarachnoid space, where there is an impediment to the reabsorption of the CSF into the venous circulation. The first disorder in which a physical obstruction is the cause of the problem is called *obstructive hydrocephalus. Communicating hydrocephalus* is the term used when the underlying problem is failure of the CSF to reabsorb. The etiology of the disorder is unknown, but the pathology is usually present at birth.

As the CSF continues to accumulate, the cerebral ventricles enlarge, the fontanels widen or bulge, and the head enlarges (see Figure 11.4). As the forehead expands, the eyes may appear depressed and a large amount of sclera shows above the iris, a phenomenon known as *sunset eyes*. Signs of increased intracranial pressure, such as pupillary changes, seizures, increased reflex responses, irritability, a high pitched weak cry, and decreased motor activity, become apparent.

Increasing intracranial pressure from bleeding or hydrocephalus can lead to downward herniation of brain tissue. Pressure on vital brain structures, especially in the brainstem, can impair respiration and other vital signs. If the child does survive, the possibility exists of permanent residual disability affecting movement, elimination, intelligence, or any body function.

Cerebral Anoxia

Lack of oxygen to the cerebral tissues during fetal development, the birth process, or during infancy can result in *cerebral palsy* and is thought to contribute to *minimal brain dysfunction*. Before birth, diabetes, toxemia, and maternal infections such as rubella may all lead to intrauterine anoxia. During the birth process, premature infants are at risk of brain damage, and complications of labor such as placenta previa or prolapse of the cord may also cause fetal anoxia. During infancy and young childhood, infections such as meningitis and head trauma can be causative factors.

The term "minimal brain dysfunction" (MBD) has been used as a "catch-all," referring to a variety of learning difficulties, behavior problems, and minor motor dysfunctions in children of average or above-average intelligence. Genetic defects as well as cerebral anoxia may be a

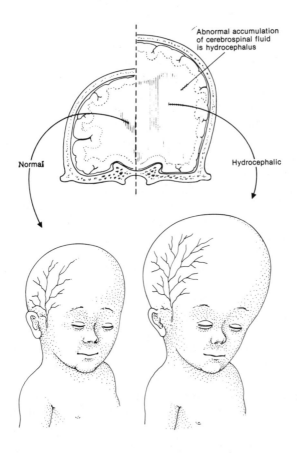

Figure 11.4 Hydrocephalus. (From William F. Evans, *Anatomy and Physiology*, 2nd ed., © 1976, p. 196. Reprinted by permission of Prentice-Hall, Inc., Englewood Cliffs, N.J.)

contributing factor, since boys are affected much more often than girls. The symptoms of MBD vary so greatly from one child to another that it may indeed seem like entirely different entities. Common behavior problems include such things as hyperactivity, short attention span, emotional immaturity, aggressiveness, and impulsiveness. Learning disabilities may be comprised of thinking difficulties, perceptual dysfunctions, and memory disorders. Motor signs involve lack of coordination and developmental lag in learning new motor skills.

Cerebral palsy may stem from the same pathological basis as MBD, that is, cerebral anoxia, but the brain damage is much more extensive.

The damage may occur in any area of the brain. Pathology that affects primarily the upper motor neurons yields *spastic cerebral palsy*, the most frequently seen form. These children have all the usual signs of upper motor neuron disease, such as hypertonicity, exaggerated reflexes, a positive Babinski reflex (see Chapter 2), retention of Moro reflex, grasp, and tonic neck reflexes. The child develops a spastic gait and may walk on the toes due to shortened tendons. These spastic effects may be seen in hemiplegia, paraplegia, or quadriplegia, depending on the area of damage. Children with quadriplegic involvement usually have speech and swallowing difficulties as well.

Athetoid cerebral palsy follows damage in the extrapyramidal system, specifically the basal ganglia. These infants have decreased muscle tone, but athetoid movements may not appear until the child is 2 years old. Then the wormlike twisting motions, especially of the distal extremities, begin. The head and neck muscles also demonstrate athetosis. Tongue deviation, grimacing, drooling, and eating difficulties are common.

The third, but least common type is *ataxic cerebral palsy*, resulting from cerebellar damage. It manifests itself in the uncoordinated movements associated with cerebellar dysfunction. There is an ataxic gait and clumsy movements of the upper extremities. Some intention tremors may be in evidence. It is also possible for children to have a combination of two forms of cerebral palsy.

In addition to the muscular effects of the disease, the cerebral damage may lead to other problems. At least half of all people with cerebral palsy are mentally retarded and many have minimal brain dysfunction. Seizure disorders occur frequently, and sensory and perceptual impairment is often seen. Some infants who are severely neurologically impaired may die soon after birth, some must be institutionalized, but many live and become functioning adults.

Infection of the Central Nervous System

The most common infection of the central nervous system in children is *meningitis*, a disease which in spite of modern antibiotics still causes death and residual disability. There are several forms of meningitis, each sharing the definition of infection of the meninges. *Viral meningitis* is the least serious type, causing acute symptoms for a few days, but soon running its course and ending without residual complications. *Bacterial meningitis* is much more serious and accounts for many infant deaths.

Bacterial meningitis may begin as a respiratory infection, and bacteria are then carried to the meninges via the blood. The bacteria multiply in the meningeal spaces and are carried throughout the CNS by the cerebrospinal fluid. Finally, organisms invade the brain tissue itself, producing an exudate that covers the brain tissue. Cerebral edema occurs, and if the process continues, brain tissue becomes necrotic.

Symptoms vary tremendously depending on the age of the child. An infant may show few of the signs that are typically present with meningeal inflammation (see Chapter 2). All you may observe is irritability, especially when being handled, lack of interest in feedings, tension of the fontanels, and high pitched weak crying.

Older children will present with fever, vomiting, photophobia, headache, seizures, papilledema, nuchal rigidity, a positive Brudzinski's sign, and a positive Kernig's sign (see Chapter 2). *Opisthotonos*, arching of the back and hyperextension of the neck, may be seen late in the disease process. A skin rash or petechiae is seen in meningococcal meningitis.

Residual neurologic deficits may appear in spite of treatment, especially if there is brainstem involvement. The child may be left with a seizure disorder, a decrease in intelligence, or perceptual and learning disorders. If the cranial nerves were affected, there may be permanent hearing loss or partial blindness.

NURSING INTERVENTIONS FOR CHILDREN WITH NEUROLOGIC DYSFUNCTION

Many of the nursing interventions used to meet the needs of adults can be adapted for the care of children. Those interventions previously covered related to sensory, communication, respiratory, and elimination problems also apply to children, often with only minor modifications. There are some nursing measures, however, which are unique to the problems of children, and these will be discussed.

Protection of Spinal and Cranial Defects

The infant with myelomeningocele requires special handling and skin care before surgery and in the immediate postoperative period to protect the contents of the meningeal sac and prevent infection. Preoperatively, and until the incision heals postoperatively, the infant should be positioned on the stomach with no clothing or bedding rubbing on the back. When the child is held (in the prone position), you must be careful not to touch the sac or put any pressure on it. Feeding is usually also done in the prone position. If there is no skin over the defect, or if it is leaking cerebrospinal fluid, a dressing is applied.

Surgery is usually performed after one day, and then routine wound care should be instituted. Watch especially for leakage of cerebrospinal fluid through the incision. The wound must be protected from contamination by urine or stool, perhaps by taping a plastic flap over the lower buttocks. Diapers cannot be used until there is good wound healing.

Protection of the head of a child with *hydrocephalus* is also an important nursing consideration. If the head is very large, the scalp may be very thin and prone to breakdown if precautions are not taken. You may be able to prevent decubiti yet keep the child comfortable if you use a foam pillow or sheepskin under the head. Inspect the scalp frequently for reddened areas. It may help to have the parents hold their child for a period of time, if allowed, to relieve scalp pressure and meet emotional needs at the same time. When holding the infant or child, always sit in an armchair so that you can rest the head on your arm, which is on the armrest. This will prevent early fatigue from the weight of the head.

Promoting Movement

It is usually easier to encourage movement and prevent complications of immobility in the case of a child than it is for adults, since children want to be active and always moving. If muscle weakness or paralysis exists, you must carry out exercises as described in Chapter 3. Evaluating muscle and joint movement is critical to determine whether the exercises that you are doing are appropriate. Your knowledge of growth and development will also help you to evaluate whether a child is capable of certain muscle functions.

Muscle spasticity, as seen especially in cerebral palsy, can be treated as outlined in Chapter 3. Parents are taught the exercises, positioning, and use of braces and other devices that can help their child. Many severely spastic children also require continuous medication. Some children may be able to attend daily cerebral palsy centers, where exercises are done as well as muscle training and various degrees of education. Assisting the disabled child to learn self-care is one of the goals of rehabilitation, and the child associated with a cerebral palsy day center will be taught to do as much self-care as possible.

Infants and toddlers with spasticity and athetosis present problems in handling. You cannot lift or position these children as you do a normal child or you will trigger spasms and flailing movements. Instead of picking the child up under the arms from a supine position and putting him or her against your shoulder, you must first sit the child up. Then lift the child with one hand behind the back and one under the legs. This extra support is essential to minimize abnormal movements.

Maintaining Nutrition

Extremely ill infants present feeding problems because they are too weak to suck or swallow properly. This is often seen in cases of head injury or meningitis. A feeding tube may have to be inserted if the baby cannot suck or swallow. If the infant can swallow but has only a weak sucking ability, bottle feedings may be possible if a very soft nipple is used. If possible, the infant should be held for feedings. This is desirable to provide the love and stimulation the child needs. Enough time should be allowed to give the baby as much of the feeding as possible.

Regulation of fluid balance is also a priority, especially in children with meningitis. A large amount of intravenous fluid may be given with the intravenous antibiotics that are used to treat the organism. If the child is vomiting, fluids are also administered to prevent dehydration. But a very real threat is the onset of SIADH (syndrome of inappropriate antidiuretic hormone; see Chapter 6). The child may already have some cerebral edema due to the meningitis; additional fluid retention will lead to water intoxication, signaled by a change in personality or level of consciousness, weight gain, and nausea.

Careful assessment of fluid balance is essential, and fluid restriction may have to be instituted. Plan how you will spread out the fluid allowance through the day. Antibiotics should be mixed in the least amount of fluid possible, as indicated in the drug literature. An IV pump may be used to make sure that only a certain volume of IV fluids is infused. If oral fluids are allowed, space them throughout the day. You can evaluate your approach to fluid regulation by asking certain questions. Does your assessment reveal fluid retention? Is the child complaining of thirst? Are the intravenous antibiotics being mixed in excess amounts of fluid? Or are the intravenous antibiotics so concentrated that they are irritating the veins and causing pain? Do the lab results reveal hyponatremia, a sign of SIADH? Continuous assessments and flexible nursing plans are an integral part of successfully managing fluid balance.

For school-aged children who are handicapped, overweight is often a big problem. Good appetites, little exercise, and sometimes boredom lead to weight gain, which can be detrimental to mobility and skin integrity. Nutritional counseling by yourself or a dietician must be done with the parents and the child, if possible. They need to learn about foods that are nutritious and filling but not high in calories, and they need help in changing eating patterns. Emphasis may have to be placed on this area of teaching, because parents with poor dietary habits themselves will find it difficult to apply proper principles for their child.

Make sure that you evaluate the parents' learning and probability of compliance.

Care of a Child with Increased Intracranial Pressure

Children at risk of developing increased intracranial pressure, for example those who have suffered head injury or children with myelomeningocele, must be assessed carefully for early signs of elevated pressure. Watch the vital signs and pupils as you do for adults. Also inspect the fontanels for widening or tension (bulging). Measure the head circumference each day, making sure that the measurements are always taken at the same place on the head. A nursing order such as "Measure head circumference QD at 10 AM, placing tape measure along top edge of eyebrows" would be appropriate.

A successful medical treatment of long-term increased intracranial pressure or hydrocephalus is the implanting of a *shunt* (a plastic tube or catheter) which drains off the excess CSF and reduces intracranial pressure.

One end of the shunt is placed in the cerebral ventricles above the level of obstruction, and the other is placed either in the right atrium or the peritoneal cavity. There is usually a small chamber or pump in the upper end of the tubing which lies under the skin behind the child's ear. CSF drains down through the shunt into the heart or peritoneal cavity and absorbs into the circulation, and the chamber is pumped periodically to keep the catheter open. As the child grows, the shunt is replaced and lengthened.

The presence of this shunt predisposes the infant to certain problems. First is the danger of infection. Infection may occur in the ventricles or in the meninges of the brain, *ventriculitis*, or *meningitis*, respectively. Symptoms of infection appear 3 to 4 days after surgery. Look for signs of redness along the superficial course of the catheter. Fever will begin, with increased pulse rate and either irritability or malaise.

The second problem that often happens after shunt placement is obstruction of the shunt. This may occur because of thrombus formation, disconnection of the catheters, or collection of debris, and it leads to a further increase in intracranial pressure. Pumping or compressing the chamber behind the child's ear helps to prevent obstruction. Include a nursing order in the care plan regarding the exact location of the chamber and the frequency and force with which it should be compressed, as ordered by the physician. Continue to measure the head circumference every day and observe for signs of increased intracranial pressure.

Positioning is of great importance postoperatively. The child is usually kept flat to avoid moving the shunt. Sometimes, though, the physician may want the head elevated to allow gravity to assist in moving CSF down the shunt. The child may be turned to all but the affected side. The catheter is placed just under the skin of the head and neck, and this skin can be damaged if pressure is put on it in the immediate postoperative period.

The parents of a hydrocephalic child need a lot of instruction before they take him or her home. They need to know how to pump the chamber on the shunt. They must practice holding and positioning and feeding the child. You have to teach them to look for signs of infection and increased intracranial pressure. But most of all, parents need reassurance about their ability to care for this infant and they need to know whom to call for help.

If the child has a noticeably large head, the parents may need a great deal of emotional support, because of the abnormal appearance, especially because of uncertainty as to what the child's capabilities and deficits may be in the future. Linking the parents up to support systems such as the clergy and local service organizations may be of great help. Parents whose child is extremely neurologically impaired may have to face a decision about institutionalization, and they may require professional counseling to help them during such a stressful time.

Controlling Inappropriate Behavior

One of the biggest problems associated with minimal brain dysfunction is inappropriate behavior, taking various forms. Although youngsters are not hospitalized for this type of problem, nurses should have some knowledge of how to work effectively with these children at times when hospitalization or health care is required for other problems. If you are assigned to care for a patient with MBD, there are a few approaches you can try that will help the child to function at his or her best and will reduce frustration and behavior problems.

A child with MBD operates best in a structured situation following established routines. Then he or she knows what to expect and what is to be done. It will be easier to get the child to cooperate with taking a bath, for instance, if a bath is always expected after breakfast.

Reduce the number of decisions the child must make, especially about unimportant things. Confronting this child with decisions about what to eat or wear or what time to play causes undue argument and friction because poor decisions are so often made and have to be corrected. Save decision making for important situations, and then guide the child into making an appropriate choice.

If the youngster is hyperactive, you should try to limit stimuli and distractions. Bringing the child to a playroom where six other children are playing boisterously would not be as therapeutic as letting the MBD child play with one other youngster with no one else around. If the child has difficulty sleeping, reduce noise in the area and remove toys or anything likely to provide stimulation.

Very often these children do not seem to hear you or they ignore what you are saying. Perhaps this is because they are so distracted by other things that they cannot attend to you. Therefore, it is best to call these children by name and secure their attention before trying to communicate a message.

Several medications have been used to control MBD behavior, especially hyperactivity and impulsiveness. The drugs used most often are methylphenidate (Ritalin) and dextroamphetamine (Dexedrine) which are both central nervous system stimulants. The reason these stimulants work is unclear. They both cause side effects such as insomnia, nervousness, and anorexia. The child must be monitored closely to make sure that food intake remains adequate and that weight loss does not occur.

Other problems of the MBD child, including all the possible learning disabilities, do not fall under the realm of nursing very often. It is usually the educator and special education counselor who handle this aspect of the condition.

Nursing Responsibilities in Child Abuse Cases

Infants and children who return to the hospital with repeated trauma may be victims of child abuse. If you suspect child abuse, you have certain responsibilities. First, any observations you make must be carefully documented. That includes the physical appearance of the child, the appearance and location of the wounds, the child's behavior, pertinent conversation, and parent–child interactions.

You are also required to report any suspicion or evidence of child abuse to designated people. Each hospital or health care agency has a protocol to follow in this situation. Generally, you should first inform the physician. If the physician is not willing to act, but you still have grounds for your suspicions, you should report to the next person designated in the protocol.

It is important that your interactions with parents suspected or accused of child abuse be noncritical and professional. If the family is being counseled professionally, you should also support the family by reinforcing positive behaviors. Child abuse is a complicated situation that requires multidisciplinary handling.

SUPPORTING AND TEACHING PARENTS OF CHILDREN
WITH NEUROLOGIC DISABILITIES

When caring for any child, well or ill, you also have a responsibility to assist the child's parents. Parents naturally become upset over even minor illness, so it is understandable that serious neurologic disorders will tax their strength and their coping abilities.

One frequently encountered parental reaction is guilt. Parents feel guilty because they did not realize their child was ill or did not take it seriously enough or did not go to a doctor sooner. If the child was hurt in an accident, they may blame themselves for not protecting the child adequately. In the case of birth defects they may also think they are at fault. You can support parents who are experiencing such feelings by assuring them that they could not predict that an illness would become serious or that a minor problem would flare up into a major one. Reassure them that no parent can protect a child every minute of the day. In the case of birth anomalies, you may have to arrange for the physician to speak to the parents to explain that they were not the cause of the baby's defects.

You can be of great help to parents if you communicate openly with them about the care you are giving their child. Explain procedures and routines, and allow parents to assist in their child's care. If at all possible, parents should be encouraged to stay with their child, to reduce separation anxiety. The more time they spend in the hospital, the easier it is for you to teach them any care that will be necessary at home. The more practice you can give them with a particular procedure, the easier they will find it to manage at home after discharge.

Parents of children who are developmentally slow should be taught the basics of growth and development. They should know what milestones to watch for and what kinds of activity their child is ready to take on (see Table 11.1). Even though a youngster is developmentally delayed, the sequence of development remains the same. A copy of a chart containing developmental milestones and respective ages can be given to the parents. You can also explain how they can assist their child to meet the expected developmental tasks.

Disciplining a neurologically impaired child is not an easy task for parents. Because of their feelings of guilt and sorrow, they may become very permissive and overprotective. They tend to give in to all of the child's demands and desires. Of course, this attitude is detrimental to the child's personality development and makes it difficult for him or her to get along with peers. If you are in a position to do so, explain the importance of appropriate and consistent discipline. The disabled child

Table 11.1 Developmental Map for the First Five Years

Age	Gross motor	Fine motor	Language	Self-help	Social
3 months	Lifts head and chest when prone	Reaches for objects overhead	Coos, laughs, squeals		Smiles, laughs
6 months	Sits without support	Picks up objects	Vocal play, wide range of sounds	Feeds self cracker	Reaches for familiar person
9 months	Crawls	Picks up small objects, e.g., raisin; thumb and finger grasp	Repetitive sounds like "baba, mama, dada"; understands "no-no"	Chews food	Plays pat-a-cake
1 yr	Walks alone (12 to 15 months)	Pencil, makes marks	Words or word-sounds (beyond "mama, dada"); comes when called	Drinks from cup	Gives affection
1½ yr	Runs stiff-legged	Builds block tower, 4 cubes	Three or more intelligible words; follows simple instructions	Eats with spoon	Asks for help in doing things
2 yr	Walks up and down stairs alone	Imitates vertical line	Two- to three-word phrases; understandable half the time; names at least three body parts when asked	Washes and dries hands	Imitates household tasks
3 yr	Goes up and down stairs, one foot per tread	Copies (picture of) circle	Phrases of four or more words; understandable three-quarters of the time; understands simple concepts like "cold, tired, hungry"	Toilet trained	Understands sharing and taking turns

4 yr	Broad jumps or skips	Cross (+) copies	Talks in sentences; completely understandable (some articulation errors); follows short series of simple instructions first..., then..., then...	Dresses self, except tying	Plays cooperatively following simple game rules
5 yr	Good balance and coordination in active play (vs. "clumsy")	Copies square, with good corners	Defines concrete words in practical terms, i.e., ball... "to play with"	Takes a bath without help	

Reprinted with permission from Harold Ireton, Ph.D., Department of Family Practice, University of Minnesota.

will never reach full potential and develop satisfying relationships if the attitude exists that the world revolves around him or her.

Parents are in a position to build the self-esteem and self-confidence of their child. The handicapped youngster often suffers from a poor self-concept because of being different from other children and not being able to succeed at many childhood activities. Parents must realize that they have to set attainable goals and not expect too much from the child. The child should be involved in activities that can be done well, and should be praised both for trying and for succeeding.

There are many community agencies that can provide information, help, and support for parents of neurologically impaired children. You can help to make them aware of and put them in touch with agencies such as the Association for the Aid of Crippled Children, United Cerebral Palsy Association, Inc., the Spina Bifida Association of America, and the National Association for Retarded Children and Adults. There may also be local organizations that can provide services and help parents to cope with caring for and raising a handicapped child.

ENHANCING GROWTH AND DEVELOPMENT
IN A NEUROLOGICALLY IMPAIRED CHILD

Children with chronic illnesses and disabilities frequently lag behind in their development. One of the reasons for such a lag may be physical maturation, or rather, the lack of it. Abilities and activities cannot develop at the expected rate if the nervous and musculoskeletal systems are not maturing normally. But physical retardation is only one factor in the situation. To develop normally, children also need a proper environment, which consists of such things as adequate nutrition, appropriate stimulation, and freedom to try new skills. Handicapped children are especially prone to limited stimulation and freedom. They may be socially isolated from their peers, limited as to the kinds of play they can engage in, and subject to different stimuli from that of a normal child.

As a nurse, you have a role in providing the kind of environment conducive to development and in teaching parents how to arrange such an environment. The first step is to assess the developmental level of the child so that you will know what kind of activities to plan. Assessment tools such as the *Denver Developmental Screening Test* are widely used and very practical. From the assessment you may discover, for example, that your 18-month-old patient is unable to drink from a cup, a task all 18-month-olds should be able to do. You may find that a 3-year-old is unable to dress herself or follow any directions. Then you can plan how to organize the child's routine and activities to bring achievement closer to the goal.

One approach you can take is to supply appropriate stimuli. For example, if a child's gross motor skills are delayed or deficient, such as standing or walking or grasping objects, you may try motivating the child to move by providing desirable items to reach for, or you can exercise muscles that are needed for those movements. Of course, these interventions will work only if the nervous system is mature enough or intact enough to enable those functions.

Another useful intervention is providing practice. Every child learns new skills by practicing them. So if you want a child to develop better fine motor skills, allow for practice in manipulating small objects, transferring objects from hand to hand, counting on fingers, picking up pencils, and similar tasks.

Behavior modification is often very successful in working with neurologically impaired youngsters, especially children with brain damage. By using principles of reward and positive reinforcement, you can help to bring out abilities that are not being used. Your 3-year-old patient who is not dressing herself, but who seems physically able, can be trained to do so by rewarding her for accomplishing various parts of the dressing procedure. Eventually she will dress herself without extrinsic rewards, simply because she wants to be successful.

Providing time for social interaction with other children may stimulate a child and motivate him or her to do what other children are doing. Children learn by imitating, whether it is adults or other children they are imitating.

You can also use play to enhance a child's development. Play should not be looked upon as just something to do when the child is bored. Even in the hospital, some time should be set aside each day for play time if the child is well enough. Play can go on in bed, the child's room, or the playroom.

By using toys and activities appropriate to the child's developmental level, you can encourage practice of new skills and refinement of old ones. Infants should have mobiles or toys hanging from the crib, and bright rattles or other toys to provide visual stimulation. By 5 or 6 months, the infant should be provided with small toys, such as balls, rings, blocks, or keys, which the baby can handle and practice grasping and holding.

One-year-olds can manipulate toys quite well and should be given practice in putting small boxes inside large ones or passing a small toy back and forth from hand to hand. They should be able to play pat-a-cake with some coordination. Toddlers are much more active and should be encouraged to play with pull toys, pegboards, blocks to stack, and balls to throw. Eye-hand coordination should be improving.

Three- and four-year-olds can ride a tricycle, draw with a pencil, color in coloring books, and play active games such as ring-around-a-rosy. They play progressively more active games if they are able, and they begin to play well in groups.

If you are caring for a youngster who lacks certain skills, such as balancing or eye-hand coordination, choose some toys or games that will give practice in these areas and work with the child. Also, select toys or games that the child can handle successfully, to reduce failure and bolster the self-concept.

Play not only helps the child to develop physically, but also to develop the imagination and creativity, to learn appropriate social roles, and to express feelings. It should be looked upon as one of your nursing interventions and should be a part of your care plan. For example, you may include a nursing order that says, "Encourage child to go to playroom at 2 PM and offer blocks, ring-toss, and similar toys that promote coordination."

By watching your patient at play, you can evaluate motor abilities, socialization, and thinking abilities. You can also use play to evaluate how well a child feels. A child with no interest in play is usually quite ill.

Concern with growth and development is an important aspect of pediatric nursing and plays a major role in caring for a neurologically impaired child. We must do all we can to help the child develop and to teach parents what they can do to help their child reach his or her potential.

REFERENCES

Bierbauer, Elaine, "Tips for Parents of a Neurologically Handicapped Child," *American Journal of Nursing*, 72, no. 10 (October 1972), p. 1872.

Chance, Paul, *Learning through Play*. New York: Gardner Press, 1979.

Cratty, Bryant J., *Perceptual and Motor Development in Infants and Children*, 2nd ed. Englewood Cliffs, N.J.: Prentice-Hall, Inc., 1979.

Davis, Gayle Tart, and Patty Maynard Hill, "Cerebral Palsy," *Nursing Clinics of North America* 15, no. 1 (March 1980), p. 35.

Gaddy, Debra S., "Meningitis in the Pediatric Population," *Nursing Clinics of North America*, 15, no. 1 (March 1980), p. 83.

Hartley, Ruth E., and others, *Understanding Children's Play*. New York: Columbia University Press, 1952.

Huber, Cathee J., and Joanna S. Dalldorf, "Minimal Brain Dysfunction

Syndrome," *Nursing Clinics of North America*, 15, no. 1 (March 1980), p. 51.

McElroy, Diane Barnes, "Hydrocephalus in Children," *Nursing Clinics of North America*, 15, no. 1 (March 1980), p. 23.

McKeel, Nancy Lynn, "Child Abuse Can Be Prevented," *American Journal of Nursing*, 78, no. 9 (September 1978), p. 1478.

O'Neil, Sally M., and others, *Behavioral Approaches to Children with Developmental Delays*. St. Louis: The C. V. Mosby Company, 1977.

Passo, Sherrilyn, "Positioning Infants with Myelomeningocele," *American Journal of Nursing*, 74, no. 9 (September 1974), p. 1658.

——, "Malformations of the Neural Tube," *Nursing Clinics of North America*, 15, no. 1 (March 1980), p. 5.

Pillitteri, Adele, *Nursing Care of the Growing Family*, 2nd ed. Boston: Little, Brown and Company, 1981.

Spitz, Phyllis, and Hannelore Sweetwood, "Kids in Crisis," *Nursing 78*, 8, no. 3 (March 1978), p. 70.

Walleck, Connie, "Head Trauma in Children," *Nursing Clinics of North America*, 15, no. 1 (March 1980), p. 115.

Appendix

Diagnostic tests

Test	Purpose	Description	Nursing implications
Skull and spine x-rays	To detect fractures, areas of calcification or bone erosion.	Anterior-posterior and lateral films are taken.	Explain that x-rays cause no pain or carry any risk. Transport via stretcher in most cases.
Electro-enceph-alogram (EEG)	To diagnose and classify seizures. To localize intra-cranial pathology.	Electrodes are pasted on scalp and a graphic recording of brain waves is produced by the EEG machine. Patient lies still with eyes closed. May be asked to hyper-ventilate for 2–3 minutes to accentuate abnormalities. Test lasts 1–1½ hours.	Preparation: Explain test to patient. Assure patient there is no pain. Hair must have been washed within 2 days. Anticonvulsants may be withheld by order of physician. Postcare: Wash electrode paste out of hair.

Diagnostic tests (*Cont.*)

Test	Purpose	Description	Nursing implications
Echoen-cephalo-gram (ECHO)	Reveals displacement of midline structures in the brain, usually by space-occupying lesions.	Ultrasonic beam is directed at the skull. Beam is bounced back off some cerebral structures and is recorded on a screen.	Explain that test is painless, non-invasive, and takes only a short time.
Brain scan	Detects tumors, blood clots, abscesses, and other space-occupying lesions.	Intravenous injection of a radioisotope is given. After waiting for it to circulate, patient is brought to the scanner, which detects cerebral uptake of the isotope. Abnormal tissue takes up the isotope in large amounts, which can be seen on a graph.	Preparation: Explain reason for delay between injection and scanning. Describe large scanning machine overhead and ticking sound it makes. Procedure is painless except for injection. Patient may have to be taken to nuclear medicine department for injection as well as scan.
Computerized axial tomography (CAT scan, CT scan)	Detects almost all intracranial abnormalities, including tumors, trauma, necrosis, hydrocephalus, blood vessel malformations, and abscesses.	Patient lies on a table or reclining chair with the head surrounded by a tight cap just inside the huge scanner. Patient must lie still for 20–30 minutes. The scanner projects images of thin cross sections of cranial tissue. Polaroid pictures are taken of the computer printouts. Injection of contrast medium may be given for better visualization. Probably the most valuable diagnostic test.	Describe size of scanner and position of patient. Explain that scanning is painless unless injection is given. Sedatives may be given to children before test to keep them still.

Diagnostic tests (*Cont.*)

Test	Purpose	Description	Nursing implications
Cerebral angiogram	To detect abnormalities in cranial blood vessels or displacement of vessels by space-occupying lesions.	Radiopaque contrast medium is injected directly into the carotid or vertebral arteries or indirectly through catheters in the femoral, brachial, or subclavian arteries. Films are taken as the contrast medium flows through the arterial and venous systems. There is some danger of a stroke or worsening of neurologic symptoms if the arterial needle loosens a plaque or vessels go into spasm. Also, possible allergic reaction to contrast medium.	Preparation: Special consent must be signed and dangers explained to patient by physician or radiologist. NPO for 4–6 hours pretest. Prepare patient as for preoperative routine. Sedative and atropine may be given ½ hour before test. Take patient to x-ray via stretcher. Explain possiblility of hot flash when contrast medium is injected. Postcare: Bedrest maintained for several hours. Check injection site for bleeding or hematoma. Pressure dressing may be in place, or a sandbag or ice pack. Check vital signs and neuro signs as ordered (Q15min–Q1H up to 12 hours). Check circulation distal to injection site if extremity is used.

Diagnostic tests (*Cont.*)

Test	Purpose	Description	Nursing implications
Lumbar puncture (LP, spinal tap)	To measure CSF pressure. To obtain specimens of CSF. To inject drugs or reduce intracranial pressure. For diagnosis of tumors, hemorrhage, multiple sclerosis, infections.	After preparing a sterile field, a needle is inserted between the third and fourth lumbar vertebrae into the subarachnoid space (below spinal cord, which ends at L1). A manometer is attached to the needle, CSF rises in the column, and pressure is read. CSF is collected in test tubes and sent to lab for culture, cytology, red and white blood cell counts, protein, glucose, and gamma globulin levels. LP is not performed if intracranial pressure is markedly increased because of danger of brainstem herniation.	Preparation: Explain that test is done at bedside. Describe discomfort from pressure, but emphasize that there is minimal pain because local anesthetic is given. Obtain special consent. During procedure: Position patient as directed by physician, either sitting and leaning on overbed table or side-lying with head bent and knees drawn up. Assist patient to stay still. Label specimens and send to lab. Postcare: Check dressing or Band-aid over puncture site. Maintain bedrest for a few hours. Force fluids to replace CSF and prevent headache. Medicate for headache if necessary.

Diagnostic tests (*Cont.*)

Test	Purpose	Description	Nursing implications
Pneumo-enceph-alogram (PEG)	To visualize the ventricles of the brain, for diagnosis of hydrocephalus, tumors, cerebral atrophy.	With the patient in a sitting position, a lumbar puncture is done; CSF is removed and replaced with air. Air becomes a contrast medium and outlines the ventricular system. This test is now done infrequently because CAT scanning has replaced it in most cases.	Preparation: Special consent must be obtained. Explain procedure after physician has told patient. Explain sitting position and fact that restraints are used because chair is rotated. Describe discomfort of LP and posttest headache. Preoperative preparation is done. Sedation is given ½ hour before test. Take patient to x-ray via stretcher. Postcare: Keep patient on bedrest with head flat to minimize headache for 24 hours. Force fluids if no nausea. Check vital signs and neuro signs as ordered (Q15min–Q1H up to 6 hours). Medicate for headache and nausea as necessary. Record intake and output.

Diagnostic tests (*Cont.*)

Test	Purpose	Description	Nursing implications
Electro-myogram (EMG)	To identify lower motor neuron dis-orders. To distin-guish between weakness related to neuropathy and weakness from other causes. To evaluate peripher-al nerve damage.	Needle electrodes are inserted into the muscle and the elec-trical activity of the muscle and supply-nerves is depicted on a screen. Muscle ac-tivity can be studied during electrical stim-ulation, during move-ment, and during rest.	Explain that needle insertion is uncom-fortable or a little painful. Explain test.

Neurologic Diseases and Patient Problems

Disease condition	Frequently occurring patient problems							
	Movement	Elimination	Respiration	Nutrition	Communication	Sensory/perceptual	Seizures	Emotional/psychological
Amyotrophic lateral sclerosis	X	X	X	X				X
Bacterial meningitis	X			X			X	
Brain tumor	X	X		X	X	X	X	X
Cerebral palsy	X			X	X			X
Guillain-Barré syndrome	X		X					X
Head injury (severe)	X	X	X	X	X	X	X	X
Huntington's chorea	X			X	X			X
Multiple sclerosis	X	X			X	X		X
Myasthenia gravis	X		X	X	X			X
Parkinson's disease	X	X		X	X			X
Spinal cord injury or tumor								
Paraplegia	X	X	X			X		X
Quadriplegia	X	X	X			X		X
Stroke (CVA)	X	X	X	X	X	X		X
Trigeminal neuralgia				X		X		

Glossary

Agnosia Loss of comprehension of sensory input; inability to recognize familiar objects through sight or touch or smell or sound; classified according to the sense involved.

Agraphia Inability to write or express thoughts in writing; a form of motor aphasia.

Alexia Inability to read or comprehend the written word; a form of sensory aphasia.

Anesthesia Loss of sensation.

Anomaly An organ or structure that is deviant from the normal; a malformation.

Aphasia Impairment in the reception, manipulation, or expression of language.

Apraxia Inability to carry out purposeful movements even though motor function is intact.

Ataxia Incoordination of muscular movement, especially referring to walking.

Atelectasis Collapse of a portion of a lung.

Athetosis Involuntary movements seen in extremities or entire body, consisting of slow, wormlike motions.

Atonic Absence of tone.

Aura A warning sensation preceding a seizure; may be visual, auditory, gustatory, or olfactory.

Automatism Action and behavior occurring without conscious purpose and thought.

Blood dyscrasia An abnormal condition of the blood elements.

Causalgia Burning pain related to peripheral nerve damage.

Choreiform Pertaining to movements that are involuntary, twisting, and writhing.

Confabulation Invention of facts, events, and details used to compensate for gaps in memory; the person is not aware of the fabrications.

Contralateral The opposite side.

Contusion A bruise; an injury in which the skin is not broken.

Coordination Smooth-working action of muscle groups as they function together in some activity.

Craniotomy An operation on and opening into the skull.

Decerebrate posture A rigid state in response to stimulation, in which the limbs are extended and reflexes are exaggerated; reveals lack of cerebral function.

Decorticate posture A rigid state in response to stimulation, in which the legs are extended and arms and hands tightly flexed; reveals lack of cerebral cortex function.

Decussation An X-shaped crossing.

Diplopia Double vision; both eyes are used but are not in focus.

Dysarthria Impaired articulation due to disorders affecting the muscles of speech.

Dyskinesia Impairment of voluntary movement.

Dysphagia Difficulty in swallowing.

Dysphonia Voice impairment.

Emotional lability Rapid changes in emotional state without apparent cause and without voluntary control.

Epileptogenic focus The exact location in the cerebral cortex responsible for abnormal electrical discharges that set off a seizure.

Flaccidity Muscular state in which there is limpness and lack of tone.

Fontanels Membranous areas between the skull bones of a fetus and infant.

Gait Manner of walking.

Hematemesis Vomiting of blood.

Hemianesthesia Loss of sensation on one side of the body.

Hemiparesis Muscle weakness or slight paralysis on one side of the body.

Hemiplegia Paralysis of one side of the body.

Homans' sign Pain in the calf when the foot is dorsiflexed by an examiner; a sign of thrombophlebitis of the calf.

Hypercapnia Excess carbon dioxide in the blood.

Hypertonic Muscle tone is increased above normal.

Hyperventilation A state in which there is an increase in rate and depth of respiration, often due to anxiety, resulting in decreased carbon dioxide.

Hypotonic Muscle tone is diminished.

Hypoventilation Reduced rate and depth of respiration; reduced alveolar ventilation.

Hypoxia Oxygen deficiency in the body.

Ipsilateral The same side.

Locomotion Moving the body from one place to another.

Melena Black-colored stools due to altered blood.

Neuralgia Sharp, stabbing, intermittent pain along the course of a nerve.

Neurogenic bladder Bladder dysfunction due to nervous system disease or injury.

Neuropathy Any disease of the nerves or nervous system.

Nuchal rigidity Stiff neck with resistance to flexion; a sign of meningeal irritation.

Nystagmus Constant rapid movement of the eyeballs; movement may be horizontal, vertical, or oscillatory.

Opisthotonos An arched position of the body seen in meningeal irritation.

Paralysis Loss of muscle function; loss of voluntary movement.

Paralytic ileus Failure of peristalsis with symptoms of intestinal obstruction.

Paresis Muscle weakness; slight paralysis.

Parotitis Inflammation of the parotid gland.

Photophobia Abnormal sensitivity of the eyes to light.

Plantar flexion Bending the toes downward toward the sole of the foot.

Postictal Following a seizure.

Premorbid Existing before the signs of disease.

Proprioception Awareness of posture and position of body parts.

Pulmonary surfactant A phospholipoprotein complex produced by the alveoli which lowers surface tension of fluid lining the alveoli.

Rigidity Stiffness; resistance to movement; inflexibility.

Scanning speech Slow speech with pronunciation of words in their syllables and pauses between syllables.

Seizure A convulsion; paroxysm of muscle contraction.

Septicemia Condition in which there are a large number of microorganisms in the blood causing fever, prostration, coma, and possibly death.

Shunt An alternate pathway or bypass created to divert the flow of fluid from one area to another.

Spasticity Muscular state in which there is increased tone and resistance to movement and tendency to sudden muscular contraction.

Stomatitis Inflammation of the tissues of the mouth.

Tentorium A fold of dura mater separating the cerebellum from the occipital lobes of the cerebrum.

Transection A cut made across the long axis of a part.

Vital capacity Volume of air that can be exhaled following a deep inspiration.

Index